HAZARDS TO THE HUMAN HEART

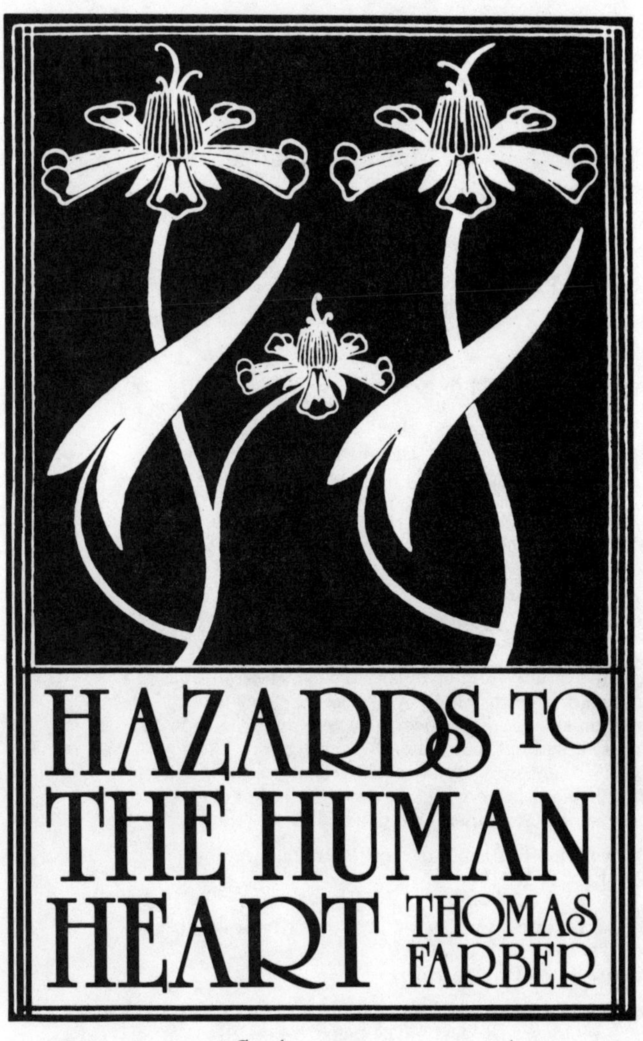

Stories of the Here and Now

E. P. Dutton New York

Stories in this book appeared originally, some in quite different form, in *Cosmopolitan, North American Review,* and *Outside*. "Whatever the Cost" was published separately as a chapbook by Donald S. Ellis/Creative Arts Book Company.

These stories are, of course, fictions. The characters, even "I," live only in these pages.

For information contact: E.P. Dutton, 2 Park Avenue, New York, N.Y. 10016

Library of Congress Cataloging in Publication Data
Farber, Thomas,
Hazards to the Human Heart.

Contents: The Mad Dog instructional league.—Whatever the cost.—The price of song. [etc.]
I. Title
PZ4.F2212Mat [PS3556.A64] 813'.5'4 79-25419

ISBN: 0-525-15424-8
Published simultaneously in Canada by Clarke, Irwin & Company Limited, Toronto and Vancouver

Designed by Mary Gale Moyes

10 9 8 7 6 5 4 3 2 1

First Edition

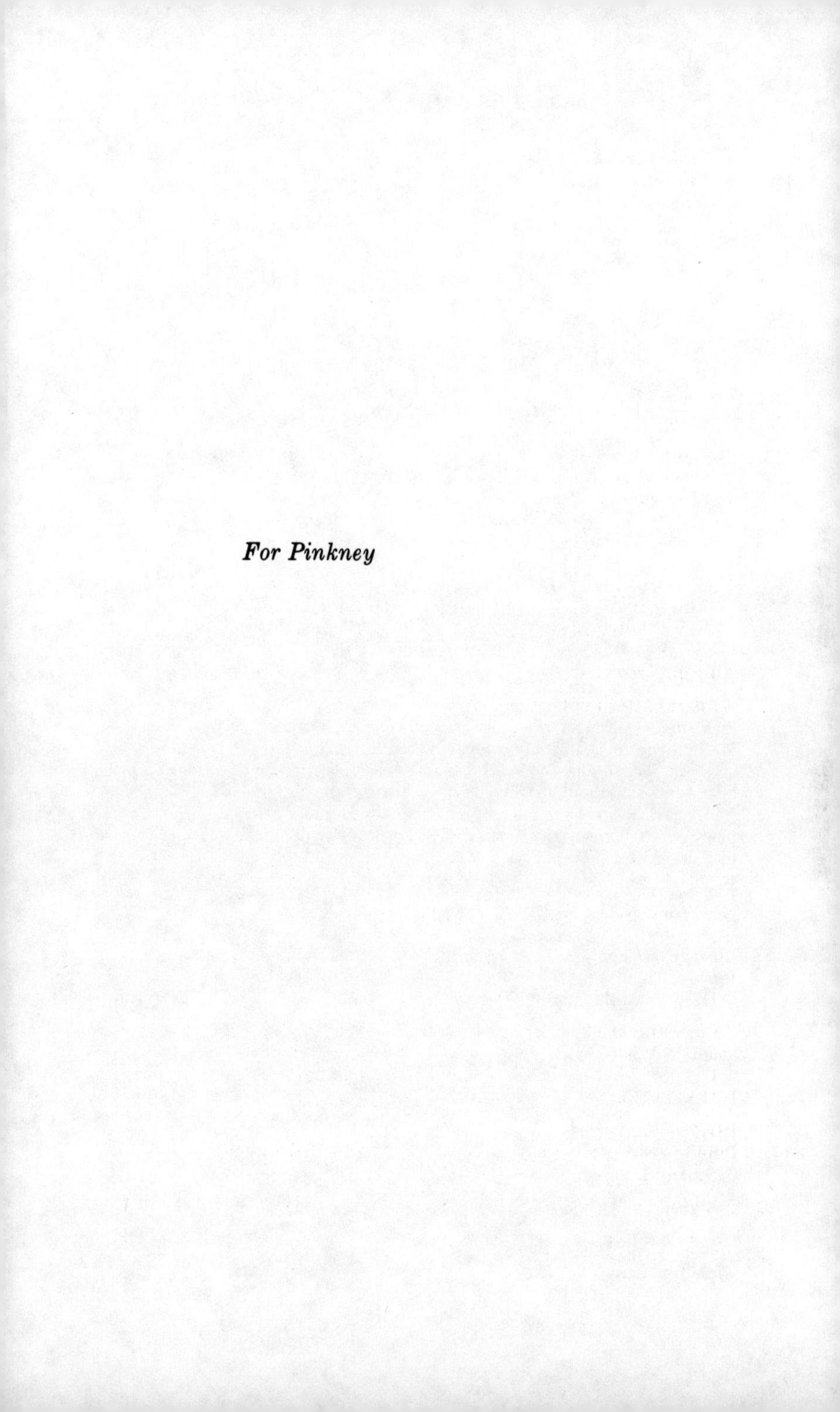

For Pinkney

The author gratefully acknowledges the generous support of the John Simon Guggenheim Memorial Foundation and the National Endowment for the Arts.

Contents

So it appears that the stickleback does not start digging because its nest-building drive is suddenly activated. Rather, the fish is engaging in what has been called a "displacement activity." Alternating between the urge to attack and to escape, neither of which it can carry out, it is finally driven by its tension to find an outlet in an irrelevant action.

—N. Tinbergen
The Curious Behavior of the Stickleback

As the proverb goes: "You don't drown in the sea, you drown in a puddle."

—Solzhenitsyn
The First Circle

There were grand passions, ordinary marriages with or without love, and liaisons both temporary and habitual, venal and affectionate.

—Ladurie
Montaillou

The Mad Dog Instructional League

"Mad Dog's back," my wife said, no trace of enthusiasm in the mother lode of her voice, a vein of pure reproach just beneath the surface. "I saw him crossing University down at San Pablo. He looks heavier, his hair is cropped, but it was Mad Dog."

"You positive?" I parried, trying in two words to express my hope that she was wrong, as well as to assert that of course I couldn't be held responsible. Christ, how much weight can two words take? I'd have liked them to convey that by mentioning his name she'd not only conjured up an image of him, but, for all I knew, had in fact caused his return. Had she not said his name, I wanted to suggest, Mad Dog might have been sitting in jail in Parrish County, Louisiana, desperate to be cut loose from a drunk and disorderly before the Feds could check out his prints and send a detainer. I could just see him sweating it out: shining on the guards, hustling the trusty, kissing the public defender's ass, swearing to the bail bondsman that he had a friend who would pay. Trying the line on anyone who'd listen, even his cellmates.

"Boy, let me tell you, if they allow me to go home I'm never coming back. I've learned my lesson. I sure hope they let me go home." Some prisoners hearing this craven bullshit shaking their heads in disgust; others venturing a smile, realizing that Mad Dog was just rehearsing—he'd con his way out.

Or, if only my wife hadn't said his name, possibly Mad Dog would have been just outside Denver, sprinting to his car for the lead pipe before surging back into the bar to crack that asshole on the head. To teach the fool a lesson: scare Mad Dog and he'll kill you. Or, maybe, he would have been in a coastal town not far north of Boston, home at last. Biting the nose off a to-that-moment belligerent unemployed teenager, only recently eager to test himself against the infamous Mad Dog.

"No question about it," my wife said flatly, straight-arming all my innuendo and speculation. "Your friend Mad Dog is back."

I don't really want to paint my wife as some kind of virago. She simply had the opportunity to say something critical, throwing in a little self-righteousness, and did so. We just weren't doing all that well together. Still partners, yes. Sparring partners. And I was looking—after what some refs might have ruled a low blow—to clip her one right on the jaw, so to speak. Forget the so to speak. I really wanted to let her have it, not so much for the way she was, but for what we now were together. At odds. Cross purposes. Out of step. All I seemed to hear from her was no. Her eyes half the time saying "I told you so." And when truces were sustained long enough to touch, maybe to make love, then her body was so sweet and rich that even as I was in her I'd become enraged to think how soon it would all be bad again.

At this marital moment, then, my wife wasn't much pleased by the prospect of Mad Dog coming around again, and I couldn't blame her. Why? Forget Mad Dog a minute. Try the times. Oh, this corpulent here and now, obliterating the past, numbing possibility, this pure present tense was on my nerves. Polyliberated northern California had by this near-terminal point in the seventies reduced itself to flu and inflation. Too harsh? Unfair? Well, true, at least the drought had ended.

There had been almost no rain for two years. Reservoirs running on empty. Hillsides brown, burnt. Water rationing up here, while southern Californians spewed water on the freeway shrubbery. Too many sunny days, no closure, no level of remove. No yesterdays. And then, finally, starting not long before Christmas, just about forty days and forty nights of blessed rain. Sewers gurgling, drainpipes leaking, ceilings staining. Green hazing the fields. Worms washed to the surface of the soil, fighting for air. And, of course, people—Mad Dog often said he'd sooner buy an

American car than trust a human being—people complaining about gray days and getting drenched. Rush hour on the Admiral Chester Nimitz Freeway in the spirit of Corregidor. Numerous "rain-caused" fatalities.

So, drought over, bricks out of toilet tanks, complaints replacing hosannas, after a winter of rain spring had come. But even as wild flowers unfurled, nothing held together for me. One weekend I turned on the tube and saw, as I scanned the spectator sports, Joe Garagiola, Curt Gowdy, Bud Collins, and Howard Cosell. Grounds for massive depression.

I'm saying not only that this was no time for visionaries, but also that opportunists had run themselves ragged. Dreams hustled into so many marketable commodities you could get embarrassed for the species. And I kept hearing all the time, from walking shards, about therapy for the whole being.

As the Bay Area continued to sprawl, people in cars creating fumes to asphyxiate themselves, having no particular place to go (and afraid I'd still be me anywhere I went), I found myself at home. Liquidating ants, the Himmler of *Hymenoptera,* though they weren't even streaming in my direction. I believed, briefly, that a pasta machine would solve my problems. I bought a pair of electric-yellow track shoes—garish is too kind a word—and wore them everywhere but did no jogging. I had the inside of the house painted white. I read junk mail. I practiced disco dancing.

In this grim period I gave much thought to the word "flu," succored by the confident brevity of such euphemism. The big words, we're told, are always short, in this case a contraction for "influenza" ("contagious . . . general prostration . . . fever and accompanying depression . . . bronchial inflammation"). In the past, hundreds of thousands died in a single influenza epidemic. For the present, forget ex-President Ford's swine flu. What we now experience is seldom lethal, merely periodic. No big deal. But, truth be told, in sunny California people get flu all the time, often can't shake it, sometimes live with it for seasons. Few Californians under sixty-five are willing to speak publicly about this, particularly once winter wanes: lack of health in fine weather suggests characterological defects.

People are always slow to accept flu in others. Several years back, I shared an apartment with a carpenter friend who was incredibly strong. He could get hit on the back by a falling beam, come home, soak in the tub, do some yoga, and be out working the next morning. When I contracted the flu—ironic understatement for overwhelming dizziness, inability to walk a hundred feet, and a sense of utter desolation enhanced by a bill for the doctor's diagnosis that I "had the flu"—I say that when I got sick my carpenter friend wasn't long on sympathy. Invisible, no stigmata: the whole business smacked to him of hypochondria and malingering. Even the most gentle souls, I've found, can be like wolves if they don't understand what you're feeling. My carpenter friend thought that what was really wrong with me was "psychological." Or that if I improved my diet, jogged more, took vitamins—all within my power, you see—I'd improve. I cannot say I cried, then, when, like an elephant downed by pygmies, he got it bad.

Flu within was matched by inflation without. Prices in real estate doubling every third year, even near-Buddhas got greedy: surely this was no time to ignore the material plane. Failure to buy into the inflationary spiral would render one a peon for life. For lives to come.

As a corollary, it seemed that the entire bottom of the economy had disappeared. Almost no one spoke of the poor, particularly of helping them (the poor themselves were strangely silent, as if ashamed, or perhaps simply awed by the widening gulf between them and the middle class). Nor was there now any such thing as junk. "Nearly new" stores prospered, marketing items "new to you"; commodities depreciated not in price but in value.

Apparent to me also was a symbiotic relationship between condominiumization and the ecology movement. Those who could no longer afford a home, but paid seventy-five thousand dollars for ownership of a small apartment, had a keen appreciation of Spaceship Earth's limited resources. If there might not be enough room in the lifeboat for possibly recalcitrant fellow citizens—the choices would be terrible—at least whales could be saved. And given the difficulties of talking to those outside one's circle, interspecies communication looked both easier and preferable.

Working myself to a frenzy as I appraised all this, I sealed my fate by deciding to stop smoking. Phones rang incessantly in my pineal gland; I was a beached fish gasping in the sun. Snorting coke to suppress my nicotine craving (manifesting itself externally in budlike excrescences which I ascertained to be yaws), I ran through a thousand bucks, quick, and contracted a mild case of megalomania. My irritation increased as I saw subordinate sections of my psyche assert their primacy. I seemed to be at school in myself, majoring in four-letter words, minoring in scatology. Though intermittently aware of what my language sounded like, I was only the more depressed, perhaps because even when nothing seemed particularly wrong, I had the sensation that the depression lever in my cerebellum had been permanently tripped. I was forever on the verge of tears.

At long last, having absorbed an overdose of my vile language, my wife succumbed. "Your fucking dinner's ready," she said one night. "It's on the fucking table."

This exchange, once articulated, stopped the present tense from moving on to another present tense, as it had been doing so remorselessly. Having remembered almost nothing for weeks, I remembered this. And, dismayed, was left to measure it against my high resolve, when we'd first fallen in love, to never—no, never!—say a sharp word to her.

But to return to Mad Dog. Why wouldn't my wife want to see him around; why would I be eager to dissociate myself from his arrival? Well, there was a day, his previous trip through, that somehow seems typical. He came over to the house while I was out and hit on my wife for some money. Knowing I wouldn't have loaned him any more, knowing it was way out of line to be asking her. When she told him no as I'd instructed her, he stormed out, slamming the door behind him so hard that the knob fell off, locking her in.

Another time he met an old friend of mine, a man about six-foot-seven. Checking him out, Mad Dog, at five-eight, now without the suggestion of a smile, told my friend he hated tall people. Or Mad Dog would walk down the street, pass some black teenagers, and mutter, audibly, "jungle bunnies." He was like that his last run through town. And finally, cursing California, saying that everyone out here was "shallow," wishing us an imminent earthquake, he left. On to a Louisiana jail, that bar just outside Denver, and the coastal town, his home, not far north of Boston.

Let me conclude, then, that there was good reason not to be glad to see him. But absorbed as I was in making and then canceling appointments with my dentist, looking for something to change if not improve, needless to say I waited for Mad Dog's call.

To defend myself in this if I can, let me defend Mad Dog, or at least flesh him out. Once we were both in Boston the night of a real blizzard, and we trudged over to Cambridge, only a few cars left on the road. As we headed for Porter Square, we watched a cab turn onto Mass Ave. and get stuck in a drift. Mad Dog walked up to the elderly cabbie and said, "Hey, take it easy, we'll handle this. Got a shovel?"

An ancient matron in the back seat rolled down her window. "Thank you very much, boys," she intoned.

"Dig you out in a flash," Mad Dog replied gallantly. "Quick as we possibly can." He began shoveling at a ferocious pace and after about fifteen minutes shouted that it was time for a try. When the cabbie, who'd been standing beside me watching him work out, headed for the car, Mad Dog said, "Wait a second, hold it. I told you we'd take care of this. Gimme the key."

Sliding in behind the wheel, he told the matron to hang on, signaled us to push, and, rocking the car back and forth expertly, finally careened onto packed snow. Leaving the engine running, getting out from behind the wheel, he said to me, "Let's go, man."

"Hey," called the cabbie. "Wait a second. Let me give you something for all that."

"No way," Mad Dog answered, deflecting the man's hand. "This one's on us. Just be more careful in the future, and take it easy."

"All right," the cabbie said. "Thanks. Thanks a lot."

"Don't mention it," Mad Dog said. Waving to the cabbie and the matron, stuffing his hands in his parka pockets, he stalked off into the black night and white snow. Another save by Super Dog.

This was the noblesse oblige of an eight-bottle-of-beer-a-day man, a self-diagnosed paranoid schizophrenic. He knew what he was doing, however, in turning down the money: who needed five, or even ten, bucks? He was getting paid for just this kind of thing, three hundred and fifty a month tax free from the state, since it concurred in his diagnosis, considering him to have a "disability." And of course with that came free medical and dental. Further, if Mad Dog chose to live more expansively, still without holding a job, he had substantial resources: shoplifting food; stiffing restaurants, particularly ones that encouraged him to run up a big tab; or, best of all, collecting from the Catholic church. This last gambit was Mad Dog's bread and butter. He'd approach a priest, make his voice thick with submissiveness and shame, and say "I'm sorry, father, but my wife is really worried. The kids are sick and we're way behind on the bills. The pressure's building; I'm afraid she's going to leave us. Can you help? Fifty dollars would really give some breathing room." Mad Dog figured he batted .666 at this hustle.

Fortunately, both disability payments and these scams were portable, so he could move around. Without obligations, he had the freedom to be gone much of the time. No one could have been more local than Mad Dog until he started wandering. Poor Irish ("resentful slobs," Mad Dog often described his kind, "resentful as a bastard"), he was raised in the small fishing town his grandfather had come over to, and for him this was the world. Playing guard on the high-school basketball team; wearing his letter jacket as he raised hell in local bars; following the Celtics and Red Sox. Always with people he knew, people he'd known all his life.

But home was also where his father, a construction worker, punched the hell out of him whenever Mad Dog (Michael, to his parents) manifested willfulness, where his mother, often as drunk as her husband, would strike him in the face with a leather belt. Though he really left home for the first time at nineteen, off to prison for car theft, Mad Dog might have been lucky to get away at all. And lucky his crime wasn't patricide. Monumentally confused by his parents' crazy blend of love and violence, Mad Dog was hard on himself and wild with others.

In high school, for instance, he attended a basketball workshop staffed by professional players. Mad Dog's teammate one afternoon in a game of two-on-two was Jim Loscutoff, an enormous man, notorious enforcer for the Celtics during the Cousy-Russell-Sharman era. On the infrequent occasions Loscutoff came into a game, the Boston crowd roared for blood.

In this particular contest, which Mad Dog wanted very much to win, he terminated his dribble near the top of the key. Unable to move with the ball now, and without hope of throwing up a percentage shot, he had to pass and waited for Loscutoff to cut to the hoop. As if there was some way for Mad Dog to get the ball to him past two defenders, however, Loscutoff simply stood in the corner. Finally, enraged, Mad Dog heaved the ball over the backboard, screaming, "Damn it, you stupid bastard, when I tell you cut, you cut." Showing surprising speed and stamina for a man who spent much of his career on the bench, Loscutoff chased Mad Dog quite a ways.

Though Mad Dog continued to be dominated by his temper, in prison he found that things could have been worse. He played third on the softball team, batted .355 at cleanup, ran the laundry, and tailored his own clothes out of standard issue. The world within the walls, closed and slow, was a community; he liked the feeling of knowing everything that was going on. No, institution life wasn't completely different from the navy career he'd often planned on, but of course in prison he never knew what crazy fucker would attack him next. And as one of the white minority inside, he had to learn much more about talking his way out of trouble, about biding his time to settle a score. He began reading psychology, the better to appraise others, to predict threats more accurately. In this he was only refining techniques he'd been shaping since childhood, when he carefully observed his parents each evening as they came home from work to see if they looked especially dangerous.

A quirk of his six-year "rehabilitative" sentence was that the time ran automatically to completion once it began, no matter what Mad Dog did. Hence, when he was paroled after two years inside, it occurred to him that if he disappeared for three years and three hundred and sixty-four days, he could come back, turn himself in for that last twenty-four hours, and tell them to shove it. Irritated with the restrictions his parole officer imposed, he picked up some phony ID and started hitching around the country, stolen official NBA basketball in the pack on his back.

Often he moved from college town to college town, becoming expert at walking onto a campus and, within hours, locating a dorm or fraternity house to sleep in. The next day he'd be playing ball at the gym. Frequently he'd stay for weeks, occasionally also auditing classes. At the University of Kentucky, which had backboards and hoops he liked, he became immersed in comparing different versions of the New Testament—King James, Gideon, Living, and Amplified. His studies carried him on to Dante, and he particularly enjoyed John Ciardi's analysis of the *Divine Comedy*.

Meeting so many people in so many environments in his travels, always the outsider, he became ever more skilled at reading and manipulating others. He took pride in this, quick to try to peg where someone was from, what kind of work he did. Hanging around students, reading their books, he knew he had far more experience to chew on than they did. Yet he was still utterly confused about the relationship between love and violence. He had the savvy to continue to run down the clock on his sentence, he could con just about anyone, he always managed to be released from arrests for petty offenses before the authorities learned he was wanted, he had even begun to gain some perspective on what had shaped him, but he was no closer to self-control.

Isolated, without the sense of place his hometown had given him, bereft, really, arguing with parents who were of course miles away, whom no one around him could possibly know, he was perpetually on the verge of rage. In Oakland one time, watching the Raiders on TV in a bar, perhaps jealous of the locals and their loud laughter, wanting some attention or recognition, the anonymity driving him insane, he felt impelled to say in a very loud voice that Kenny Stabler was just an overrated piece of shit. Left-handed shit, for that matter. Mad Dog won the fight—escalated first to a lead pipe, then ran faster—but he couldn't help himself. He longed to go home. Was dizzy with so many strangers, so many miles.

Finally, the clock on his sentence still running, he returned. Finding his younger brothers out in the yard, he was just calming down when his mother came out of the house.

"I knew you were back," she screamed. "I just knew it. What are you doing, you criminal; haven't you screwed up your life enough? Now you're messing up your brothers."

"Hey, ma, don't talk like that," Mad Dog said. "Especially in front of the kids. I'll be gone soon; I'm just here to see them. It's been a long time."

"Not long enough, you good-for-nothing. You can stay away forever, for all I care. Get out or I'll call the cops."

"I heard her talking like that," Mad Dog once explained as we downed Irish coffees. "I saw her making me the evil heavy with the kids. Telling them I was a no-good slob. Shit. I knew what I was. Out of my mind most of the time. Half in the bag the rest of the time. But she didn't have to run me down like that. See, she had dominated me for years. She blinded me twice with that leather belt. She's sick, but very very bright. You can really dominate people when you're that sharp. And women are like that. Deviant."

"Devious?" I asked.

"Whatever. I mean you have to keep 'em in check or they'll spin these crazy webs. They're totally unpredictable. You can never tell what they're going to do next. Fortunately, most of them you can control by letting them do what they want, because basically they're not very aggressive people.

"But my mother, she was something else. She scared my moron father, and that's a fact. Anyway, there I was at home again after being away so long. It was really something to see my little brothers. I just about raised them, since she and my father were stinking blind drunk every day. I made dinner, sewed up their torn clothes, got 'em off to school, everything.

"So, there she is again, and I couldn't take it. I gave her a shot, broke her cheekbone. Then I guess I got a little crazy. Smashed all the windows in the house. I'll tell you, though, next time I saw her she was totally different. Totally polite. You know, if you really beat someone, wicked brutal and quick, a surprise, you stymie them. You take a piece of their life."

This, then, is the Mad Dog my wife wasn't eager to see around, the Mad Dog whose call I was waiting for. My wife wasn't wrong, of course, but she wasn't living inside my skin. She was, however, close enough to see me playing the soundtrack from *Rocky* for hours every day, earphones on my head, arms raised high as I jogged in place. A winner! And she did see me sitting at the breakfast table, grinning as I read in the morning paper that the federal government was financing sex changes for indigents. Nodding my head knowingly, as if another theory had just been confirmed.

Soon Mad Dog was stopping by nearly every afternoon. He'd come walking down the street sipping a "Tall Boy" can of Schlitz wrapped in a paper bag. Liquid brunch under wraps. Always he was careful to have me step outside immediately, afraid that if my wife saw him too often she'd find a way to set me against him. Usually we'd go play pickup half-court basketball near campus with the other unemployeds and unemployables, three-on-three or four-on-four. Or maybe we'd go one-on-one, Mad Dog showing me another move Cousy taught him or criticizing me for not protecting the ball better on the drive. Urging me to run with him in the mornings to build up my stamina.

He was a good teacher, carefully explaining a complex move, breaking it down into components, working steadily and quietly on each with me until he felt it was time to try the whole. Day after day he was methodical and persistent, if too quick with praise. But he wanted me to learn, "to reach my potential."

"With your height," he often said—I'm around six-one—"there's nothing you can't do in this game." And it seemed true. After a while he had me jumping out from a low post to take a pass, setting, and going way up in the air for my jump shot. Strength from underneath, soft touch on the release. By the time I thought I had it down he was waving a broom in the air in front of the hoop to force me to put more arc on the ball. And, amazingly, my shots were going in, the net giving that beautiful soft swish on the clean ones.

Despite the beauty of what I was learning and my rapid progress, both Mad Dog and I were of course begging a simple question: what sane man would be getting deeper into basketball—not to mention giving it the best energy of each day—at age thirty-three, just the time when most court heroes switch to tennis or concede to paunch, if they haven't long since. When the prospect of being clobbered from the blind side or twisting an ankle outweighs even the possibility of dunking the ball. But there I was, the hoop my Bodhi tree, a self-confessed space case my guru.

As a player Mad Dog was very good, no question about it, especially when he didn't flip out. Which, unfortunately, happened regularly. Someone wouldn't be passing to him. The game would get senselessly rough. There'd be too many big men on the court—Mad Dog brooding about how great he could have been at six-three—clogging the middle, and no rule in half court to make them move around, opening space for more agile players. Or he'd become despondent to think of how it was when he played full-court ball on a hardwood floor, banking shots off a glass backboard.

Not untypical was the day he simply quit playing defense altogether during a game. No one on his team noticed until they saw the man he was supposedly guarding drive in for a second uncontested basket. When his teammates, not unreasonably, asked him what he thought he was doing, Mad Dog exploded.

"Look, this maniac is clobbering me. I'm not going to get hurt just because he's out here."

"Then sit down and let someone take your place."

"To hell with that. Tell this fool to sit down. He doesn't know anything about the game."

"Fuck. What an asshole."

"Who's calling me an asshole? Come on, say it again and see if you can still remember your fucking name. Scumbag."

"Hey, man, be reasonable, will you? If you don't want to play why don't you be cool and sit down?"

"You be cool. You sit down. The man can't play ball. Get him off the court. I'm staying and that's all there is to it."

Though Mad Dog was not all wrong, since the man he was covering had no body control, of course he could have switched assignments with one of his teammates. Instead, enraged, he'd destroyed the game. It was, sadly, also true that he'd missed his first five shots. Had they gone in, he might have put up with almost anything for the chance to keep shooting.

Despite such explosions, when it occasionally all came together he'd be jubilant—achievement and community so clearly defined. Hitting his jump shot. Or faking it, waiting till he had his man up in the air, then driving all the way, sometimes finishing with a stutter-step underhand layup to rub it in. Or he'd hurry back on defense, intercept the ball, and set up a back-door play with sharp passing.

Such moments waned too quickly, however, and there was no film crew recording it all for posterity. Players could and did praise each other, one might sit for an hour after the game savoring what had happened, but it was often bad feelings that lingered longest.

At the least, the rules of the game were a source of endless conflict. Without the penalty free throws of organized basketball, there was little reason not to foul. The injured party could only stop play and take control of the ball. Further, in the absence of referees, disagreements over even these barely punitive calls were often resolved by sheer obstinacy and verbal violence: a man would insist he was right and hold up the game until he got his way. Such infantilism, surprisingly, was motivated less by a desire to win than by the endemic court affliction—a hopeless disparity between ability and self-image. Since many a player was in his own mind an undiscovered or former star, it followed that no one else could possibly know as much about the game. Certainly not the other players, obviously bums.

Much of this on-court autism and assertion of infallibility derived from the maxim, "I shoot, therefore I am." Though aware that the great professional basketball dynasties subordinated individual virtuosity to team play, many pickup players seemed incapable of passing the ball once it came into their hands, as if it were thence irresistibly drawn up toward the hoop. The need here was not simply for the visible success of scoring but for a conclusive demonstration of dominance. To teammates, the message, "I'm the best, therefore I'll do the shooting"; to opponents, "Do you really think you can possibly stop me?" Strangely, off court many of these atavists—their hungers harkening back to an era well before the arrival of the hunter-gatherer—were reasonable men. The game, however, brought out the very worst in them. In most of us.

"I'm going to tear that asshole's larynx out," Mad Dog said one day as we walked off the court. He was speaking of a ball hog who had kept yelling for Mad Dog to pass to him. I could find no fault with Mad Dog's sentiment, particularly since we'd lost a close game that had been a hybrid of rugby and UN debate.

No doubt this depiction of the game's negative qualities is overdrawn. There was also much banter and camaraderie, savoring of skill and idiosyncrasy, respect for ability, and even gentility. Courtliness! Especially when one became a regular and, very important, played when there weren't too many men waiting. Then at least there wasn't so much competition for scarce resources, the court less a behavioral sink. Yet life in the game was often nasty, brutish, and—if you lost—short, a Hobbesian microcosm that only confirmed Mad Dog's world view.

Frequently all this would become too much for me, though I had nowhere better to go, really, and I'd swear it off. Only to return within a few days. At such times I was also avoiding Mad Dog, his possibly contagious violence, and the feeling that he was pulling me down. This was unfair, but he'd sense my distance and stay away for a little while. Knowing the weight he could impose, he never wanted to outlast his welcome. "I'm a loudmouth," he'd say. "Fucked up. That's the way it is."

On the court, in any case, he'd found his niche. Everyone

knew him; it was acknowledged that he could really play the game. The court his community, he worked hard to ingratiate himself to the other regulars, particularly if he'd recently flipped out. As if in atonement, he'd then avoid argument—to general applause—the only catch being that he'd go to any extreme to agree with everyone, shining them on, flattering them, whatever was necessary. LSD, he told me, showed him that he should be less violent. But when his pendulum swung away from anger, often he could only play the fool, diminishing himself to make others feel life-size. Deeply skeptical of most people's motives and capacities, wanting desperately to count the court regulars as his friends, knowing the mayhem he could inflict on them if he only chose, Mad Dog alternated between blind rage and obsequiousness.

Life on the court, of course, hardly encouraged candor. I think of the time I watched Mad Dog play an attorney one-on-one. The man was good and incredibly competitive, going again and again to his two strong shots, taking no risks, concentrating on the game, grinning inadvertently each time he beat Mad Dog on the drive. He was, nonetheless, carrying an extra twenty pounds around his waist, had been smoking far too much, and was well past thirty. Mad Dog—basketball his vocation, always in training—had much more stamina.

Unlike the attorney, Mad Dog called no fouls, slacked off on defense, eased the pace. Threw the game, giving it away as one might when playing a child, only pretending to go all out. It was a convincing performance. Exhausted but still pushing himself on, the lawyer was elated when he won, gracious, if a bit condescending, in victory. Mad Dog, after all, was clearly lower class, uneducated, unemployed.

Why did Mad Dog let him win? Because he perceived that if the lawyer lost he'd be furious with himself, that soon his anger would be transmuted to an intense dislike of the man who'd forced him to confront those extra pounds, all the cigarettes, the years that had passed. The lawyer was a Princeton graduate—major league in the game of life—but had so little self-knowledge, and so primitive a faculty of generosity, that I stared at his hands to see if he had opposable thumbs. It was when playing this notable that Mad Dog, on his friendship-at-any-price kick, preferred to lose.

This lawyer was only one of the regulars. There were also some psychologists, teachers, and counselors, and a number of college students. Lots of men between jobs. About half a dozen ex-cons. A minister. A former city manager. A jazz drummer. And a radical doing a Marxist analysis of a local police force. Mad Dog snorted in disgust when he heard this player's politics and quickly forgot his no-argument program.

"You poor sap," he shouted. "You want to help people? You're dead wrong. Want to change the world? Just remember this: ninety percent of the people in this country are mean, dumb, selfish, and jealous. I know; I've been all over, every state and Canada. You've read too many books. The people you want to help would fuck you over in a minute if they could. As for criminals, I say shoot 'em, shoot 'em all. I believe in those police vigilantes. You know why? Because up until a couple of years ago I was a total maniac, pure and simple. If they had wanted to stop me they'd have had to kill me. No way around it."

As if to add emphasis to his point, that same evening in his skid-row hotel Mad Dog confronted a pimp who was making noise in the corridor. Mad Dog had warned him before, more than once sat up in bed shouting curses and threats after being wakened in the middle of the night. But this time, now also enraged at being underestimated, he reached for his lead pipe. When the pimp finally staggered off, bleeding badly, Mad Dog walked downstairs to the pay phone in the lobby, dialed the police, and reported that he'd been assaulted.

Phenomenally anxious, as usual, after losing control, still "wired as a bastard" the next morning, Mad Dog paced back and forth, reliving the confrontation, unable to shake the feeling that he might just as easily have killed the pimp. True to form, he decided that it was time to leave town.

More than a month passed before he showed up again, walking down the street, basketball in his pack, wearing his made-to-order "Don't Scare Me or I'll Pipe You" T-shirt. Apparently he'd been in Reno the whole time, visiting an old girl friend. His story took some time to unravel, however, not only because he was knocking back the six pack he'd brought with him, but because he took out his ball and played catch for a half-hour with the neighbor's five-year-old. Patiently explaining how to throw and hold it, steadily encouraging him, gauging the improvement judiciously, a little disappointed when the boy finally ran off. Like me, the kid had "lots of potential."

But Mad Dog really had important news. "Listen, man," he said, "my girl and I are dead in love. No shit. We already consider ourselves married. Fuck the government. We're going to love each other and raise our kids. That's going to be that. Nothing can separate us. But none of this modern shit. There are two roles: man and woman. Read the New Testament. Check it out. Everything has to be orchestrated by the man. You can't give women an inch. They're basically warped. Man sets the boundaries. Give them limits, they can function. But you have to be fair, too; you owe them answers. That's how it is."

If Mad Dog's philosophizing did not augur well for marital bliss, on the other hand he was looking pretty good. That he had chucked his favorite lead pipe seemed a fair indicator of emotional gain. Unwilling to go completely naked in this vale of tears, however, he carried with him a can of police Mace. "Just a squirt guaranteed by the manufacturer to blind you," he said. "But only temporarily."

If Mad Dog was making progress of sorts, so was I, and no longer by crawling on my psychic belly, whimpering. Or by shooting baskets. I could, however, regress to rage merely by wondering what was causing the improvement. Or, put another way, by wanting some explanation of my misery. Too much white sugar? Capitalism? Asbestos poisoning? Cocaine madness pure and simple? I seemed in any case to have stopped smoking (was that it?) but allowed myself an occasional hit, like a former junkie skin-popping. I did sit-ups each morning, ate vitamins C, E, and B-complex. I stopped drumming my fingers on the dinner table.

Late one night I went out for a walk. The city was strangely still: no dogs barking, not a car moving, no rock music carrying in on the west wind. Perhaps, for a change, no rapists at work. One of my cats wandered out to see what I was up to, wanting some company. When I picked him up he made a point of complaining, but I didn't mind. I'd been pretty peevish myself.

As I headed back inside, my wife was just finishing her day. Snails cleared from the garden one last time. Cod-liver oil—emergency treatment—on the roots of an ailing plum sapling. Cats inspected for fleas. Though I felt on the verge of satori, compared to the recent past, the change must not have been visible: I walked by, and my wife stared at me as if I were lucky not to be wearing a straitjacket.

I browsed around the house, letting my mind wander, trying to remember the part of myself that had once felt a kinship with so many others, that had held all our hopes in common. I couldn't locate the precise feeling, but at least it had occurred to me. I'd find it again, another time. I got into bed, turned off the light, looked out at the balmy darkness. I slept.

In the morning Mad Dog came by. He said he was getting ready to take off, going to Reno to pick up his girl, then on to Boston. Home again. We hadn't seen each other for almost a week. I was playing much less ball. It was just too piggish, and—the hideous truth hurt—I was shooting poorly. I'd also had enough of Mad Dog for the moment. He understood: long since, he'd had enough of himself.

We drank some beers, marveled at how well Yastzremski was hitting, and shared fears that the Red Sox pitching staff would fall apart in August. "Look for me on the tube when they play the Yankees," Mad Dog said. "Third-base side." Then he smiled, opened his pack, and handed me a present. It was a very expensive walnut plaque inscribed with my name, and, under it:

> Most Improved Player, 1977–1978
> Mad Dog Instructional League

I knew without asking that he'd ripped off the trophy store near his hotel. But of course he'd paid, somewhere else, for the engraving. And the idea was his own. "From one madman to another," he said, and we both laughed. Laughed like a bastard, as he'd have put it.

Whatever the Cost

for Chester Aaron

Here was a man who thought his bride beautiful. If in the first weeks of their marriage he was, not surprisingly, consumed with desire for her nakedness, a corollary of the passion they shared was his awe at how fine she looked in even the simplest clothing. Studying her as if with new eyes, he was utterly overwhelmed by the gentle curve of her breasts under a tight sweater, the long line of thigh and shank in Levis, the cascade of hair over a plain blouse's white collar. Oh, she had her flaws, he knew, but he no longer really saw them. Not even her crooked teeth.

Opting for a simpler life, they took up residence on a small farm soon after the wedding, and dressed accordingly. Even so, catching sight of his wife bending to weed the garden or stretching on tiptoe to reach an apple, he marveled that the most functional clothing was never less than a foil for her beauty. He praised cotton, gave thanks to denim, no longer disparaged synthetics.

Of course the honeymoon came to an end. Giving her a down parka, he soon had cause for regret: what kept her warm also obscured, no, obliterated the lines of her figure. He couldn't stand it, tried to take the parka back. "You look like the Michelin tire man," he said. He was equally dismayed when she discovered sweat pants and began to wear them every day. She bought several pairs, dyed them various colors, even made some of velour. "I don't think they look good on you," he told her. "I don't care if they're functional. I know it must sound foolish, but can't you just humor me?"

Though he saw her in parka and sweat pants until he cursed winter, thought of moving to Hawaii, he was solaced when they occasionally had reason to dress up. She'd go into the closet, rummage through her thrift-shop collection of dresses, choose a pair of heels, and emerge looking absolutely elegant. Torn between admiration (wanting to see her this way forever) and lust (eager to undress her immediately), he'd remind himself what a beautiful woman he'd married.

As they prepared for a friend's party one night, he suggested that she wear a black velvet suit he found particularly becoming. "I can't," she said. "I have no boots. I gave them away; they were worn out." A long silence followed her words. He was remembering that, years before he met his wife, he once gave his lover a very expensive pair of handmade shoes. He'd been working in the city then, bringing home good money. Now he had to watch what he spent.

His mind continued to wander. Did his wife know about those handmade shoes? Of course not, he told himself. How could she? He would never have mentioned it. Or had he?

"I don't really need them anyway," she said, interrupting his thoughts. "I'd almost never get to use them here."

"Maybe not," he responded, "but I just decided to buy you a new pair."

"You shouldn't; they'll cost a lot." She laughed. "You'll regret it."

"Hey," he said. "I'm going to do it. And that's that."

Several months later they flew to New York to visit some friends. Accustomed now to country life, he was both startled by the city itself and truly amazed at the clothing people were wearing. Even the men were into high fashion, dressed fit to kill. His roommate from college, for instance, had forty suits, countless monogrammed shirts, and twenty-five pairs of shoes. As for the women, obviously they spent much care and money on what they wore. In fact, only by reminding himself that he was just passing through town did he avoid feeling somewhat drab in his Abercrombie and Fitch Viyella shirts and baggy corduroy pants. No, the country squire look just didn't cut the mustard in the Big Apple. He was also chagrined to find that friends of both sexes admired his wife's velour sweat-pants creations, asked where she'd bought them.

One afternoon he suggested they go looking for boots. Since they were staying in SoHo, they began in the Village and walked down Eighth Street, where there were supposed to be some good buys. His wife saw one pair that interested her, but he found them inadequate. "They look cheap," he said. "If we're going to do this, let's do it right."

The next day they walked all the way up Fifth Avenue until they reached Saks. Though he was already tired, this trek proved only the beginning. Over the next several hours they tried Ferragamo, Bendel's, Bergdorf's, I. Miller, and Bloomingdale's. Rendered nearly catatonic by the crowds, the array of merchandise, and the prices, he persisted because he had in mind boots that were very simple, of obvious high quality—"classical," he kept telling his wife—but hadn't seen any. She, meanwhile, tried on a pair of green suede spike-heeled boots with turquoise embroidery; lace-up ostrich-skin ankle boots with detachable spats; and, completely forgetting their mission, pumps of silk crepe de chine.

As the afternoon ended they sat drinking coffee. "Sorry," he told her. "I have a headache. I'm exhausted. Let's call it a day." They were walking back toward Fifth Avenue looking for a cab when he stopped abruptly at a store window. His wife, who'd gone ahead several feet, turned and rejoined him. "Now this is what I meant," he said triumphantly. "Wasn't this worth waiting for?" The boots were both chic and austere, extraordinarily beautiful. And, he noticed, no prices were indicated.

The shop was small but luxurious, the chairs incredibly comfortable, the clerks dressed for disco dancing. As his wife tried on first one pair of boots and then another, his head began to nod. She poked him on the arm. "Do you like these?" He did, but, looking around at the displays, suggested she try several others. As his eyes closed again he heard the cashier tell a woman he'd seen trying on a pair of iridescent leather flats that it would come to one hundred and fifty-one dollars and thirty-three cents. Dear God, he said to himself, what will boots cost?

"Those are two hundred and ninety dollars, plus tax," the clerk told him as his wife walked back and forth in front of the mirror in a pair of burnt brown Spanish-style riding boots with contrasting trim. "They're designed by our experts here and then crafted in Milan. Each boot, of course, is handmade."

"Well?" he asked his wife as she sat down, beaming. "Should we get them?"

"They must be incredibly expensive," she said.

"Let me worry about that. Do you want them?"

"Who wouldn't? But do you really think they're worth it?"

As he took out his BankAmericard, hoping he hadn't already exceeded his credit limit, the cashier explained that they also had a selection of boots for men. "No thanks, not today," he replied. Not unless you take used Adidas in trade, he said to himself.

"Happy?" he asked his wife as they walked toward Fifth Avenue to find a cab.

"Yes," she said, "but I hope you won't regret it."

"Don't worry, I won't," he replied. Yet, even as they stood on the curb waiting for the light to change, he was translating the price of the boots into house payments (one and an eighth) and shaking his head. Come on, he told himself. This is something special. She'll have the boots for years. I'll love seeing her in them.

Nevertheless, he couldn't help thinking that it was a lot of money. Of course she'd hardly pressed him to spend it. He'd made the offer in the first place; he'd suggested that they go shopping; he'd found the store. Still, it was a hell of a lot of money for a pair of boots. No question about that. She knew it too. He wondered, accordingly, if she'd feel she owed him something for such a wonderful gift. He looked over at her, noticed her crooked teeth. No, probably not. She'd assume, not unreasonably, that he'd done what he wanted to do.

He kept thinking. Though the whole venture had been his idea, wouldn't it be something if there were a quid pro quo he could now expect from her that would somehow defray the expense? But what? He laughed to himself. What indeed?

The light changed; they moved with the flow. She took his arm, boots in a plastic bag dangling from her left hand. He kissed her cheek. What a beautiful woman, he thought. Really, what could he ask for? And, if he were in fact able to find some way to broach so delicate a subject, what would she think the boots were worth? Could he, for instance, ask her to stop wearing sweat pants? No, probably not, not now that so many people had admired them. Too bad. Too damn bad. The boots would have been cheap at the price.

They walked on, her arm still in his, people streaming past in both directions. It began to drizzle. The sweat pants would certainly have been worth it, he told himself, worth every last penny. What a shame. Well, that was that. So what else could it be? And then, not only consoled but starting to grin, he remembered the down parka.

The Material Plane

What's bothering Cecille? Why isn't she cleaning the ranch house the way she always does, sweeping the floors, washing the dishes, straightening up after the twins? Why didn't she make Gabe's sandwiches this morning at dawn before he saddled up? Why didn't she bake apple pie yesterday, so there'd be some left over this morning for Gabe to take up to the high country? She knows how much he likes it. And why hasn't she fed the chickens, collected the eggs, milked the goats? Cecille knows that only work will make the ranch pay, Gabe's said so a thousand times, but still she's just sitting in the living room, Bach suites for cello on the stereo, looking out the window at the rain. She should be putting on her boots and foul-weather gear, but instead she's trying to imagine Boston, where she was headed the day she met Gabe.

There may be more direct answers to explain what's bothering Cecille, but one might begin with tansy ragwort. A tall weed with yellow flowers, tansy is pretty enough but, for ranchers, a persistent problem. When cattle are crowded on land or minerally deficient, they eat tansy and can be fatally poisoned by its alkaloids. Tansy is hard to eliminate, but it can be controlled. Even as Cecille sits staring out the window, the fields of tansy are under attack by striped orange and black cinnabar-moth caterpillars.

Though voracious, however, the cinnabar can't keep up with the tansy's awesome seeding. Yet it happens that sheep seem to be able to eat tansy without danger. By methodical cross-fencing, enough sheep can be contained on any given section of pasture to both clear out the tansy and keep down poison oak, bracken fern, and greasewood. Meanwhile, if properly constructed, the fences may also deter coyotes, thus saving lambs.

This isn't, as they say, the half of it. If you're into progressive pasture-management techniques the way Gabe is, you take cognizance of what's called the nitrogen cycle. Consider a legume like clover, which fixes nitrogen through nodules in its roots. Bacteria in the nodules put that nitrogen into the soil. As the clover develops, it provides enough nitrogen to make rye, fescue, and orchard grass produce well. If sheep are then grazed intensively, they not only crop the grasses, which thrive on being driven hard, but their manure—more nitrogen!—keeps the clover and grasses growing. This means winter pasture growth; just what the ewes need when lambing. Richer milk. Healthier lambs. Ultimately, not only is nothing lost, but a self-tending system of ever-greater plenitude develops.

But the fencing, the fencing. Much of the expense and labor comes from trying to make the fence coyoteproof. Strychnine now banned, a four-foot swath of woven wire is topped with two strands of barbed wire, then sealed at the bottom by a two-foot wire apron. The fence route is leveled into a road, the slope of the hill cut back to prevent easy leaps over the barbs. Whenever he can spare the time, there Gabe is, fencing and cross-fencing. Scuttling uphill on foot, fast, looking—pudbar in hand and construction helmet on his head—like a Spartan hoplite, four sticks of dynamite and some nitrogen fertilizer tamped into a stump below. About to go off. The explosion waits, waits some more, and finally crackles like a thunderclap through the background drone of the flies. A cloud of dust rises and, slowly, settles. But already Gabe is back on the huge D-8 Cat (from any distance no more than a toy, cute, and yellow like tansy), feet pumping the two brakes, hands flying from Johnson bar to blade-control lever to clutches as he surges forward, backs, wheels, and screeches, forcing his way down the slope at an impossible angle. Time passing, other tasks cared for, the seven-foot treated fir posts will be driven in with a rammer on the back of a John Deere. The wire will be laid out, stretched, and tightened with the Cat. Stapled, hog-ringed, and, at long last, done. One step toward improving the ranch.

Gabe, you see, has a dream. He wants to make this place show a profit, and then he wants to buy another. Two, in fact. One for each of his young sons. He doesn't want to end up like his father, too broke to go into town for a meal, owing bills at the feed store. Fences in disrepair, animals sick and lost. Drinking whiskey to start the day. Botching everything, finally getting his skull staved in by his own horse. No, at thirty Gabe's willing to work for what he wants, unwilling to let anything stop him.

To make the ranch pay, Gabe goes flat out all year round. Doing mechanical work in the winter when getting around the hill country becomes too treacherous, tearing down and rebuilding engines; putting out hay to help the stock resist the stress of cold, frost, and occasional snow. Lambing in January, calving in March. Doctoring and marking by the end of May. Shearing in June. Preparing for market, haying, fencing, and logging through the dry summer and fall. Doctoring the cattle again, and weaning calves, before the rains return.

Consider just the logging, one task of many. Always short of cash because he reinvests the money from the sale of lambs and yearlings back into his flocks and herd, Gabe logs as much timber each year as he can. Setting out early in the morning, always, to avoid the heat of the day, chain saw slung up on his shoulder, three-foot blade cushioned on a folded burlap sack, gas can, oil jug, and ax in his free hand, Gabe trudges up through alder, poison oak, myrtle, and cedar, looking for trees to fell. Picking one, deciding where he wants it to land, studying curves in the trunk which suggest that it will split and shoot back when cut, checking wind direction and force, Gabe grunts as he jerks the starter cord on the saw. He places his undercut, knocks it out with the ax, and steps around the tree. Sawdust now shooting back from under the blade, foul-smelling water pouring out of the white ("piss") fir, Gabe slices into the rear side, perhaps making additional cuts to stop the trunk from pinching the blade. And then, moving away quickly, he watches as the tree tilts, creaks, breaks, rips, and crashes.

For a moment, saw stilled, there's quiet. Sunlight filters down, air full of the myrtle's aromatic smell; the northwest wind soughs through the branches. But Gabe has his rhythm and, gear gathered, is already moving on. Later he'll return to trim the trees and haul them out with the Cat, then buck the logs into standard lengths for the mill. All this is hard and dangerous work. Stories of loggers being maimed and killed are common. But for Gabe, timber is money, and money buys him time to increase his stock and finish the fencing.

A little more than six years have passed since the day Cecille first drove up the four miles of unpaved road to the ranch in Gabe's battered '52 pickup. Hitching through the Northwest, in no hurry at all, she was on the first leg of a trip cross-country from San Francisco to visit her brother in Boston. She was twenty then, about to begin her sophomore year of college, and tired of feeling too well protected. She'd traveled, even to Europe, but always with her parents or as part of an organized group. Her parents had objected vehemently to her plan to hitchhike alone, but she'd told them, quietly, that she could take care of herself. Her confidence was confirmed in the first four days on the road: rides came quickly, one after another; everyone was friendly. She stayed overnight with some musicians in Eureka, camped with a family in a VW bus on the beach in southern Oregon. The proprietor of a roadside café offered her a job as a short-order cook.

The morning Cecille met Gabe she'd taken a ride inland with some longhairs. They left her off in a small town which, it seemed to her, was in the very middle of nowhere, flat green country with clusters of dairy cows standing under isolated shade trees. She'd walked on past town about a mile when Gabe drove up and stopped. He didn't say a word, simply leaned over and punched the door, hard, throwing it open. Cecille climbed in, smiling and saying thanks, but Gabe only shook his head as she tried several times to close the door. Then he leaned past her, grabbed the handle, and slammed the door shut. Cecille's initial impression of Gabe was of disparate parts: his straw cowboy hat, shocks of red hair pushing out from under; his silence; his long legs folded under the steering column; and his right hand, nails filthy and broken, skin scarred. An old man's hand, Cecille thought, though Gabe was obviously in his early twenties.

As they drove along, his silence was so profound that she couldn't think of a way to break it. She failed even to ask him how far he was going or what road would connect with a major highway. In another context, hitchhiking alone, she might have found such silence menacing, but Gabe simply seemed remote. After about ten miles, as he approached a crossroads grocery and post office, he said, "This is as far as I go." It was high noon, hot. Not a car in sight. Cecille began to gather her pack and jacket.

"Have you ever done ranch work?" Gabe asked, looking straight ahead out the dirty windshield.

"No," Cecille said quickly, assuming now that she'd misread him, that he was making some kind of advance. "I'm on my way to Boston to visit my brother. Then I go back to school."

"People learn a lot on a ranch," Gabe said, still looking straight ahead.

Cecille couldn't control her laughter. He had to be putting her on, she thought. The taciturnity, the avoidance of eye contact. It was surely a parody of rural style.

"People learn a lot in school," she said, still laughing.

"Maybe," Gabe answered, now looking toward her but not quite meeting her eyes. "Maybe. But I'm getting a ranch going. I'm looking for someone who can cook and clean and garden. Fifty dollars a month and room and board."

Cecille laughed again. This really would be a story to tell her family and friends. "Woman's work, is that it?"

"That's right," Gabe said, apparently missing her sarcasm.

"Well," Cecille replied, thinking it had gone far enough. "I'm not looking for work right now. I have plans."

"Ever see a ranch?" Gabe asked, as if she hadn't just rejected his suggestion.

"No."

"Why don't you visit one before you make up your mind?"

Cecille looked down the road. Still not a car in sight. Sun hot and high. "How far is it?"

"Four miles."

"You promise to drive me back down?"

Gabe nodded, and, before Cecille could say anything else, shifted into first gear and headed up the dirt road, a plume of dust streaming out behind each rear tire. Finally they approached the ranch house, which sat tucked in a hollow, a creek flowing behind it past corral and barns.

"This is beautiful," Cecille said, surprised. But Gabe seemed not to hear her, or to speak right past her words.

"I'm alone here. I need someone to help."

"For the woman's work?" Cecille asked, again sarcastic, thinking that her friends would never believe someone his age could be so out-of-date.

"That's right," Gabe said, apparently missing, or ignoring, her tone.

Weeks later, Cecille learned how Gabe's father had died, that his mother had run off years before, and that Gabe had been in the merchant marine, traveling all over the world, so that his country manner was at least partly a matter of intent. But that afternoon she had little to go on. Marveling at the beauty of the land, however, she decided to stay for several days. Another adventure. Yet, strangely, Gabe did nothing at all to encourage her, going off on horseback without inviting her, saddling up as she watched him, without a word about when he'd return. It was nightfall before he came in, clearly exhausted, only nodding his head to acknowledge her presence. Breaking out a can of franks and beans with a look of reproach, as though he'd expected her to have dinner prepared.

While he'd been gone that afternoon, Cecille had inspected the ranch house, startled to see how dirty it was, the absence not only of order but of any softening touches. He really did need someone, she thought. She'd also walked out to the barn and corrals and had seen the dogs.

"Why do you keep the dogs like that?" she said when they sat down to eat.

"Like what?"

"Chained up."

"So I know where they are."

"All day?"

"They're here to work. They're not pets."

"But why do you need so many?"

"Two for sheep, three for cattle. Two growing up to replace the ones that get hurt."

"I think it's horrible," Cecille said, self-righteously.

"I'm running a ranch here," Gabe responded. "I don't have much time to play."

When he fed the dogs later that night, however, Cecille was surprised to see him let them off the chain. Was he doing it for her? He spoke quietly to them, teasing them as they swirled around him, a kaleidoscope of black and white, shooting up at his face over and again like porpoises. Seeing Cecille watching, Gabe said, "They're Border collies. Purebred. Expensive. And it took a lot of time, too much time, to train them. But they're good dogs."

That night Gabe showed Cecille a room, empty except for a mattress on the floor, a bare bulb hanging from a cord in the ceiling, and gave her a few blankets. No sheets, no pillow. Cecille had trouble sleeping, heard two owls hooting back and forth for hours, woke frequently. In the middle of the night she opened the window and looked out. There was no light in the sky, the fog in low, air moist and absolutely still. Past the outlines of the myrtle, oak, cottonwood, and maple she could just make out the barn roof's sharp slope.

When Cecille came down in the morning Gabe was gone and didn't return until late afternoon. Though she had considered staying several days, she was piqued by his lack of attention.

"I thought you were going to drive me to the road," she said, feeling slightly foolish as she heard herself.

"Sorry. I had trouble in the high country."

"You should have taken me along. I'm a good rider."

"We'll see, then. I have to go back up tomorrow."

The next morning at six he knocked on her door, and by the time she came down he was outside, sitting on his horse and holding the reins of another. This was more like it, Cecille thought. For nearly an hour, dogs running on ahead, they climbed slowly through the ground fog, sun finally breaking through. As they came over a rise onto the high south-facing prairies, they saw several elk. Cecille was elated.

"I wish I had my rifle," Gabe said.

"Why would you want to shoot them?" Cecille asked.

"I don't hunt," Gabe said, "but elk destroy the fencing. They don't even try to jump the fences sometimes, just plow on through. You don't know this country or what it's like to run a ranch. You can't imagine how much work they cause. They're beautiful, but I wish I'd brought a gun."

Cecille knew that she should say something more, that no one should kill such animals. They were wild, free, had to be saved. But what Gabe told her made sense, given his perspective. At least he wasn't glad to shoot them. That was in his favor. As they rode on, time and again Gabe sent the three dogs into the brush to drive out the groaning cattle. "Way 'round now," he'd shout, and the dogs would surge off in a wide circle to get past the cows and calves and stop them. Once this was done, Gabe would call "get in behind" to bring the dogs back, cursing under his breath if they were slow to respond. Then he and Cecille would canter along to another area. Finally they drove the stock they'd gathered down to the corral behind the ranch house.

Though she'd loved the riding, Cecille was exhausted and quickly depressed both by Gabe's obvious intention to continue to work and by the corral itself. The bare muddy ground and weathered gray planks had escaped her notice the day before, but now she began to appreciate the relentless progress of the pattern. The main corral fed into a small corral, which opened into a holding pen, which in turn funneled into a narrow walkway down which Gabe drove the cattle with an electric prod. Cecille thought of pictures she'd seen of Bull Connors and the marchers in Alabama.

Gabe forced each animal into the inverted V of the squeeze's bars. The opening behind clanged shut each time, and, as the cow or calf lurched forward, the front gate caught it at the neck and shoulders. Tongs Gabe placed in the nostrils jerked the head up. And then, depending on what he decided had to be done, Gabe cut ears and tagged them, branded, vaccinated, wormed, fluked, castrated, dehorned, checked for pinkeye, and, finally, with another clanging, released the terrified animal to a holding pen. Her stomach turning, Cecille forced herself to stay. But Gabe was too busy to notice, his bloody hands reaching for drench gun, hoof trimmer, prod, branding iron, worm gun, knife, Elastrator, syringe, dehorner. "I'm sick," Cecille finally shouted and ran up to the ranch house, sure she'd leave in the morning.

She didn't leave, of course. Perhaps because Gabe made no advances. Cecille couldn't even take it as a sign of respect; he just didn't try to sleep with her. And her admiration for his drive and skill was growing. The next day she rode with him again and watched him separate a bull from some cows. Cantering through the pasture, rocking easily in the saddle, Gabe brought his gelding next to the bull and guided him—both animals now thundering along—flank to flank, buffeting the bull over and again, forcing it yard by yard up the hill. It was a dangerous job, done well, but Cecille gave Gabe no praise, still annoyed by his apparent lack of concern about whether or not she'd stay.

That afternoon she watched him fix one of the gelding's shoes, taking the hoof and putting it up on a broken axle that functioned as a makeshift stand, deftly tearing off the shoe, cleaning out mud and rot, cutting back the nail with rippers, and filing the hoof smooth. Then, having straightened the shoe on the anvil, Gabe turned his back to the gelding's head, bent over, took the hoof through his legs, and supported it on his knees. The gelding shifted his weight restlessly, tossed his head. "Way, way, come on now," Gabe said softly. Towering over him, the gelding pulled back. "Take it slow, come on," Gabe said. Grunting with exertion, he drove eight nails into the shoe, cut off the ends, and filed them down. Cecille was moved, the same way she'd been when Gabe let the dogs off the chain the first night. He was incredibly gentle with the gelding. The work was rough, often cruel, Cecille thought; but Gabe wasn't.

The next day she began to clean up the house and cook the meals. She started by washing the walls and floors, finally, after a week, feeling ready to paint. Each evening Gabe came back filthy, fed the dogs, and sat down to eat. "You're on the payroll," he'd said that first evening, "but spend as little as you can. You'll have to put in a garden. I'll slaughter an animal for some meat." He seemed pleased that the house was cleaned but said nothing at all about the painting, as if he simply tolerated it. When Cecille gave him the bill for the paint and brushes, he raised his eyebrows and stared but didn't stop her. Merely left the suggestion that she was doing it for herself, not for him.

Cleaning out an upstairs closet about a week later, Cecille came across a box of books. There were many paperback Westerns, and, to her surprise, the collected works of Joseph Conrad.

"Whose books are those?" she asked, when Gabe came in that evening.

"Upstairs? The Westerns belonged to my father."

"Who read all the Conrad?"

"Me."

"Why such an interest in him?"

"I wanted to get away from home. And I did. I joined the merchant marine when I learned that Conrad had left Poland, a landlocked country, and become a sailor. I figured if he could do it, then I could at least make it fifty miles to the coast."

Cecille was elated. No one at home would believe it. A cowboy who read Conrad and had been to sea!

Soon Cecille had been on the ranch a month, having written her brother several times to say she'd been delayed. As weeks passed, she was aware that it was almost time to return to San Francisco to get ready for the fall semester. On the whole, she was pleased with herself. She knew she'd helped Gabe, she'd learned a great deal about ranching, and she'd have incredible stories to tell. She hadn't reached Boston, but she'd get there next summer, or maybe even at Christmas. The only thing that bothered her was that she and Gabe hadn't made love, hadn't kissed or even touched, for that matter. She just couldn't figure him out.

Then one day she got chilled swimming in the creek. It was her own fault. She'd been taking a dip late each afternoon, both to bathe, since the shower was broken, and in the hope that Gabe might see her as he returned to the ranch house. Still she was irritated by his apparent lack of desire for her. There was no sun that particular afternoon, and even as she got dressed she was shivering badly. By the time Gabe came back she was in bed. He felt her forehead, made her some tea, covered her with extra blankets. She tossed and turned all night, but each time she woke she saw Gabe sitting in a straight chair beside her bed, dozing, long legs stretched out before him, bits of hay in his red hair.

She came into his room one evening not long after she recovered. It was transformed now that she'd cleaned and painted it. Walls white, floor bright blue, small throw rug on the floor, wild flowers in a vase. She got into Gabe's bed and stayed the night.

"Why did you make me wait so long, and why did I have to come to you?" she asked when they woke in the morning. "You know you're my favorite cowboy."

"I guess I'm shy," Gabe answered.

"Is that really it?" Cecille said, only half joking, thinking that maybe he just hadn't wanted her, hoping to be reassured.

"I guess I don't like fast women," he said. He was smiling; he had his arm around her.

"You know, the trouble is that I think I believe you."

"There's more."

"What?"

"I wanted to see if you really liked the ranch."

"I should sleep with the ranch, then."

"I'm serious."

"You're strange. Or maybe just straighter than straight. I thought your type was dying out."

"It probably is. But before I'm gone, let's make love one more time."

About two weeks later, Cecille told Gabe she'd have to leave soon to arrive at school in time for registration. By now she didn't want to go but had no idea what Gabe was thinking.

"Of course there's a lot to learn at school," Gabe said, grinning. "Then again, there's a lot to learn on a ranch."

"So?"

"But if you stay and live on the ranch like this, people will talk."

"I want to stay. Let them talk."

"No," Gabe said quietly, "I don't think that's the way to go about things around here."

"Then what?" Cecille said, about to cry, thinking Gabe was telling her to leave.

"Well, I think we'd have to be married. I think that would pretty much shut people up."

Gabe didn't want a big wedding, no ceremony at all, really, so they settled on a justice of the peace in the small town where he'd picked Cecille up on the road. They took no honeymoon, however: Gabe said he just couldn't leave the ranch with market time coming right up. A month later Cecille rode by bus down to San Francisco, startled, once there, by the crazy variety of life, the light, the laughter, the numbers of people, the choices of ways to be. She was sorry Gabe hadn't come, but she returned to the ranch full of energy, thinking of the many changes she'd make. Friends would visit, her parents too. They'd all love Gabe. She'd get a car, so as not to have to depend on Gabe's schedule. And she'd find a stereo. She did in fact receive a stereo from her brother as a wedding present, but friends came seldom and usually stayed no more than several days. Always Cecille felt abandoned as they drove off. As for the car, when her parents gave her their old station wagon she got the feeling that Gabe was displeased. She asked herself repeatedly if she wasn't mistaken, but it was true. Gabe didn't want her to be able to leave the ranch whenever the spirit moved her. He considered the ranch his world, got uneasy when any part of that world wasn't under his control. This was something that called for understanding, Cecille told herself. Gabe's mother, after all, had run off. In time Gabe would see; he'd learn to trust her.

Now that she had the car, however, she decided to visit her sister in Seattle. She urged Gabe to come, pointed out that the neighbors' son could do the chores for a week, but Gabe insisted he had no time to waste. He could still get some logging done, he said, before the heavy rains began. When Cecille responded that she'd have to go herself if that's how he was, he simply refused to discuss it further. Clearly he felt betrayed. Cecille made the trip, finally, driving away from the ranch in a rage, but she was gone less than a week, worrying about Gabe the whole time. When she called from Seattle, she told him she was sorry. He didn't make it easy for her to apologize.

As that first year passed, she learned more and more about ranch life. How to start the pickup—putting a heel on the floor starter as you gave it gas with the toes of the same foot—was the first lesson, then how to drive the tractors. With Gabe's help she put in an enormous garden and carefully planted rows of marigold and mint against insect predators. She began baking loaves of bread each week, and pies. She learned how to repair engines, sharpen tools. She got goats and ducks for milk and eggs. She canned and dried fruit and vegetables. When lambing began, she learned how to put her hands deep in a ewe's womb to help a breech birth, and soon had ten motherless lambs—bummers—feeding in the living room. She kept so many bummers alive, in fact, that Gabe made no objection when she insisted on keeping one, marking it with red dye so it wouldn't be carted off to market by mistake. The lamb followed Cecille around like a pup, even went swimming with her in the creek.

Cecille would not, however, help Gabe butcher the animals they consumed themselves. She knew it was inconsistent—she ate lamb or beef almost every day—but she couldn't, not after the time she watched Gabe slaughter four wethers. He put them in the front yard that morning, closed the gate, and shot two, a bullet apiece. Once more Cecille had to admire Gabe's skill. Then he raised them off the ground with the tractor lift and quickly bled, beheaded, skinned, gutted, and halved the carcasses. He returned to the front yard, took up his rifle again, and dropped the third wether. The fourth, now alone and smelling blood, surged from end to end of the yard. Waiting patiently for a good target, Gabe finally fired. Blood spurted out of the wether's mouth, but, crazily, it came right at Gabe, then broke past him across the front porch and down the road. Cursing, Gabe chased and at last downed it, slitting the throat as he broke the neck. The sun eased through the clouds; yellow jackets gathered on the wheelbarrows teeming with innards. Though she knew Gabe hated what he called "false sentimentality," Cecille began to cry.

Perhaps she was overwrought because she was pregnant. For months before the twins were born, in fact, she wondered if she'd been right to marry Gabe, and now to have his children. Her parents had come up to meet him and see her new home, but, though they'd said how beautiful it was, clearly the life seemed harsh to them. Her father, a doctor, was an opera buff, her mother a singer of lieder music. For them the ranch was a place to visit, but no more. When Gabe, trying to be polite, expressed sympathy that they had to live in a city, her father corrected him, going on at length about the riches of urban life. Inviting Gabe, pointedly, to come and see. Sometimes, reading the weekly letter from her mother, thinking of the concerts her parents were going to, of the incredible mix of her parents' friends, Cecille would find herself ground down by the practicalities of the ranch. And by Gabe's monomania. Everything had its function. Animals were raised to be sold or consumed. Fruits and vegetables too. Pups that didn't show promise were shot. And, it occurred to Cecille, she too had her place on the ranch. To cook, to clean. And to breed.

She chastised herself for such thoughts, felt disloyal to Gabe. He'd never dissembled; he was just as he presented himself. A man building up a ranch. His aspirations had moved her, she'd responded to his dream. More, she knew how vulnerable he was, the shame he'd felt for his father, how he'd suffered when his mother ran away. But understanding Gabe didn't always help. Still she could find no way to make him compromise. She'd been certain when they married that she'd be able to enhance the gentleness that was clearly in him, to get him to ease his pace. But now, with her help and presence, he seemed only more driven. And life on the ranch was all on his terms, his personal preferences buttressed by the demands of 2,000 acres, 750 animals, and loan payments. Cecille began to feel that she could argue with Gabe but not with the whole damn ranch. She kept the bummer lamb, built hummingbird feeders, put candles on the table at dinner, bought linen napkins, to insist that not everything had to be functional. She did all this but felt as though she was only losing ground.

During her pregnancy, sometimes scared of what she had set in motion, she'd laugh bitterly to herself. Visitors found the ranch so romantic, but they knew little of the reality. Of course there was the branding, the castrating, the butchering, the endless dirty and dangerous work. But beyond that, seeing the ranch as remote, visitors failed to understand how exposed it was. At the least, much of Gabe's land was unfenced, and in any case all fencing was porous. Elk and bear flattened it at will; nothing could keep all the coyotes out. More, even on horseback with the dogs, working the heavy timber and brush of the high country, Gabe could never be certain he'd gathered all his stock. Was it just the inevitable four percent wandering around up there, or had someone been rustling?

Reinforcing this sense of permeability, and far more intrusive, were the hunters. Both Gabe and Cecille dreaded deer season. Some hunters moved with caution and respect for land not their own. But others, crazily overarmed, drinking heavily, crossed property lines at will. Skidding and winching up impossible slopes, eroding prairies and rutting out roads, loaded rifles pointed out the windows. Eager for their quota, often shooting even in a heavy fog at any sound of movement. Gabe could post the land, of course, but legal proceedings suggested only wrath incurred, and cattle were simply too easy to pick off. Ultimately there was no obstacle to determined hunters. Gunfire echoed in the hills. Resting in the afternoons, Cecille often pulled the pillow over her ears, but there was no escaping the sound.

Sometimes even the language of the ranch country drove Cecille wild. At first the economy of gesture, composure, and taciturnity seemed quaint, almost comic, to her, but slowly she sensed that it was all structured for an avoidance of direct requests and refusals. No one wanted to give offense. A grudge might develop, a barn might be burned. Cecille knew that Gabe was comfortable with the circumlocutions, found protection in them. And she often loved him the more as she watched him talk to other ranchers with an abiding reserve that Shane or the Virginian would have grudgingly admired. Yet no matter how much it suited Gabe, this was also the mode of people who had something to lose. No one, she thought, was "up front." Women on ranches nearby spoke with her frequently, were generous and helpful, but remained neighbors. No more, if no less.

Just before the twins were born, another rancher's stray cow was hit by a car on the road near the house. Though the animal was suffering, Gabe refused to shoot it until he could reach the owner and get his approval. Cecille listened, hour after hour, as the animal groaned in pain. She begged Gabe to put it out of its misery. Surely, she argued, the man would understand. But Gabe waited a day and a half.

Once the twins were born, Cecille had little time to wonder if she'd chosen the right life. Between caring for the boys and her endless round of chores, questions were a luxury she couldn't afford. Spring, summer, and fall, she and Gabe went flat out, and winter never seemed long enough for a real rest. She made one trip each year with the twins to visit her parents but had little energy for exploring the city.

As the boys grew and she watched Gabe initiating them into ranch work, she began to feel that already they were not hers. What could they know of the world she'd come from? Perhaps, she told herself, they could spend time with her parents when they were older, summers, or even go to boarding school in San Francisco. It would be a battle with Gabe, of course, and she was glad such a possibility was years off. Meanwhile Gabe still drove himself, though by now the cross-fencing was finished, tansy under control, stock increasing each year. Other ranchers, doing less well, took vacations in winter when things slowed down, hired foremen, but Gabe was looking for another ranch. Since Cecille met him he'd gone no more than the fifty miles to cattle auction.

The fall the boys were five they went off to school. Suddenly, after years without a moment to herself, Cecille had time to daydream, to simply look around her without trying to get something done. She began to relax, no longer feeling that she was always behind, struggling to catch up. Hungering for something new in her life, wanting to see the world outside the ranch, she signed up for an ecology course at the regional junior college fifty miles away, planning to make the trip two nights a week. Far from supporting her in this, however, Gabe argued that the hundred dollars for the course was a waste of hard-earned money, not to mention the cost of gas and wear and tear on the car.

"But this is something I want to do, Gabe," she said, struggling to control her anger.

"Nobody gets everything they want."

"You do," Cecille suddenly shrieked. "You do."

"Lower your voice," Gabe said. "The boys can hear."

"Let them. It's about time they heard me say something. You wanted another ranch, so you put us in debt all over again. No questions asked. You wanted another tractor, you bought it. Did you ask me about that? You wanted to increase the flocks again instead of keeping the money. Who asked me? When is it ever not what *you* want? And now you tell me, the first time I've done something like this, that a hundred dollars is hard earned? I know what it took to get that money. What do you think I do around here all day? I know it was hard because I earned it. Over and over and over again. And don't you dare tell me I didn't."

Cecille shouted these last words at Gabe's back as he slammed the front door behind him. He said nothing more about her taking the class, but neither did he apologize. If anything, she thought, he was harder than ever, less open, more set against any manifestation of her autonomy. If she hadn't had the car her parents gave her, she was sure, Gabe would have made it impossible for her to go.

At class she met students who worked in the mills or at various small businesses in town. Their wages were small, they had no hope of better jobs, but to Cecille they seemed remarkably free from care. Despite Gabe's silent opposition and the long drive, she looked forward to each class. Only twenty-six, she'd begun to think of herself as an older woman, no longer young in any case, in part because of the twins. Her classmates, however, simply assumed that she was more or less like them. Several men at school asked her to join them for drinks, and, though she begged off, she was flattered. Gabe had for some time seemed to take her for granted, and the few males she saw at the ranch—other ranchers, the cattle buyer—were always ponderously careful to treat her less as a woman than as Gabe's wife. She felt younger each week the semester passed, laughed more. Maybe, she thought, she could even loosen Gabe up a little.

One day when the twins were off at school, Cecille stepped out on the front porch and saw a hunter only several yards away. Bowie knife and pistol on his belt, rifle in hand, wearing fatigues and an army jacket. Beside him was a dead buck, clearly underage. She felt the hunter watching her as she looked at the deer. This kind of thing had happened before, many times, and Gabe liked it no more than she did. Over and again she'd seen Gabe check his temper, forcing himself to be civil, waiting until the hunter left his land. But this time Cecille couldn't do it.

"That buck is too small," she heard herself saying. She knew Gabe would be furious if he learned.

"Oh, I don't know about that," the hunter said easily, meeting her eyes. "I'd say it's okay. Wouldn't you, now that you think about it?"

Cecille heard the threat but was so angered by the very presence of the hunter that she was unable to stop herself. "No," she said. "Count the points for yourself."

"Oh, that," the hunter replied, grinning. "That's nothing we can't fix." He pulled out his pistol and fired four times, blowing the antlers to bits. "There now," the man said, holstering his gun. "No more problem."

"But I saw it," Cecille said, her ears still ringing from the shots.

"Well," the man responded, "I guess you might have made a mistake."

"No," Cecille said, "I didn't make a mistake." Scared, she went inside and locked the door. Finally she heard the man drive off.

Late that afternoon, walking the bottom land on her way to check the apple trees, she heard several shots back toward the ranch house. More hunters, she thought. When she returned from the orchard, passing the barn, she saw a bull on its side, still alive but slowly bleeding to death from a gunshot wound. There was no way, Cecille realized, not so close to the house, that the shooting could have been accidental. The hunter must have returned to teach her a lesson. Cecille went inside, got Gabe's rifle, placed a shell in the chamber, and walked out toward the barn. Putting the muzzle against the bull's head, she pulled the trigger.

She was still there, sitting beside the bull, when Gabe came down from the high country. She'd thought of lying to him, but when he reached her she told him about the hunter and what she'd said. She waited for him to explode, but he just nodded his head as if he'd expected as much. As if she really had no place on the ranch. Still silent, he walked over to the shed, backed out the small tractor, and hauled the carcass into the barn.

For several days not a word passed between Gabe and Cecille. She stopped baking bread, made no pies. Then the winter rains began in earnest, and her depression deepened. It would be cold and gray for months. She thought of visiting her parents but had no energy for the trip. She'd gone through it all too many times. Packing up, going to the bus station, riding all those miles. Seeing her parents, having to answer their questions, knowing they always worried about her. Being overwhelmed by the city. Only to return to the ranch to find Gabe the same, herself the same. Each morning she packed the twins off to school, but each day she spent more time letting her mind wander. She stopped canning and drying fruits and vegetables. She had to force herself to milk the goats. She missed one class, then another. Days passed, a week, but still Gabe didn't speak to her. He was freezing her out, she thought, and she was turning to ice. Was this what Gabe's father had done? Was that why his mother had run off? Cecille stopped cleaning the house. Dishes piled up in the sink. There were no clean clothes. The twins complained. Still Gabe said nothing. Without a word, finally, he did a wash but left the dirty linen napkins in the hamper.

Late each afternoon now, when the twins came home, Gabe returned from whatever work he was doing, got them into their rain gear, and took them out with him. He began to make them breakfast and supper. Each day, watching this, Cecille spent more time thinking. When Gabe rounded up the cattle from the high country, bringing them down to the corrals, she played Bach cello suites on the stereo to drown out the sound of the cows and calves calling to each other. Did the cows know the separation was final, she wondered. Did the calves know it was time to die?

Cecille felt herself losing control but could think of no one to ask for help. She gave up altogether the idea of going to class. What was the point? She had endless bitter imaginary arguments with Gabe, screaming at him to say something, to leave the ranch, to come with her to San Francisco. To show her some love. Convinced, suddenly, that he would try to sell her bummer lamb, she closed it in the barn. She sat for hours in her workroom, returning again and again to the day Gabe picked her up on the road. The longhairs who had given her a ride that morning. The spot where they'd left her off. The feeling of being in the middle of nowhere, clusters of dairy cows standing under isolated shade trees. The heat of the sun. What would have happened, she kept wondering, if she hadn't taken the ride. If she hadn't gone up to the ranch. If she hadn't stayed. What if she'd continued on? Where would she have gone? Who would she have met? Where would she be now? Would she be different? How? Who would she be? What would Boston have been like?

Something to Protect

Early February in northern California, cold and gray, storm winds gusting in from the south, hard rain battering the premature plum and cherry blossoms. Fallen reds, whites, and pinks carried off on rivulets. False spring, a bad time for the blues, but Mike's trying hard to bite the bullet.

Mike: a laid-back accountant, witty, unfailingly courteous, scrupulous, an eligible bachelor. And sick at heart, head over heels in love with Suzanne, who has now been gone four days—and three nights, damn it!—without calling him. He can't stand what he's thinking, tries to get hold of himself, says out loud, as if making the sounds will help, "I'm climbing the walls." If only it weren't raining he could go to the ocean, sit in the sun, something, but instead he's alternately berating himself and building an airtight case against her.

"What kind of slob are you?" he asks himself. "She just wants some room to set things straight. She said it was too soon for commitments. She loves me." True, true, but the heart weeps: she's with her former love, who's come back to town for a few days. "I have to see him," she'd concluded. "He's miserable, he says he has nothing to live for now, that I owe him a few days."

"Do you think I shouldn't?" Suzanne had asked, but Mike had said nothing, both wanting her to make her own decision and seeing some good reasons why she should go. Cut the ties once and for all. Explain how things were. Say good-bye. Forever. But what was she doing for four days? What could possibly stop her from calling? What kind of person would not call? Mike is chain-smoking now. Her brand. He's going insane. What wasn't she doing?

Four days by the phone, waiting. Finally, mind reeling, Mike goes to see Tony and Doreen. Angry at himself for needing to be cheered; certain Suzanne will call the moment he's out the door; wild at her for what he's going through—what she's putting him through.

"She went to Big Sur to see Jeff?" Doreen asks, her voice incredulous.

"I didn't know she was going there," Mike replies miserably. "She got up Friday morning, having finally decided Thursday night that she should see him. Then, an hour after she takes off, she calls and says she's driving down to his place at Big Sur, that he's already there. She said she'd be back as soon as she could and that she loved me. I was pissed, but I didn't want to make a scene, particularly not on the phone."

"Well, at least she called," Doreen says. Mike groans. They both know that in the past she's disappeared from more than one lover to go back with Jeff. Mike's spent a month with her, they've had only good times, but now he wonders if it all was no more than an interlude in her ongoing melodrama with Jeff. *Was?*

"You'll have to get it settled as soon as Suzanne comes back," Tony says.

"That's precisely what I mean to do," Mike answers, his voice thin with anger. "We've gone too far, way too far, for this kind of crap."

"She may not want to hear it right off, though, particularly if Jeff's been screaming at her," Tony observes.

"That's the way it goes, then." Mike cracks a knuckle, then another. "I can't take this any longer."

"You know," Tony begins a moment later, coming back from the kitchen with some beer, "when I met Doreen we had an incredible six weeks together, and then we both went east for Christmas. We planned to meet in New York after the holidays. She was coming down from her folks' place in Maine, stopping in Boston to spend a few days with her sister. I spoke with her when she was with her folks, and then I tried her in Boston. I kept leaving messages with her sister, but she seemed to have no idea who I was. Finally she told me Doreen was staying at the apartment of the guy she'd been living with before we met."

"David," Doreen adds.

"Right." Tony rolls his eyes. "I'll never forget what's-his-name. Anyway, by the time Doreen arrived in New York I was wild. At the airport I told her she had to decide. Either we were going to continue what we'd begun and settle for that—at least for the foreseeable future—or we could separate."

"I only went to see David because I wanted to make sure he was all right," Doreen says. "You can't spend years with someone and then just cut off all contact."

"That's what I thought when Suzanne told me Jeff was back in town." Mike likes Doreen's point. "I figured they had things to settle."

"Maybe so," Tony replies, "but it depends on what stakes are being played for. I may have been wrong, totally wrong, but I don't think so. David was still in love with Doreen."

"I was worried about him," Doreen explains. "I didn't want him to do something crazy."

"Florence Nightingale," Tony says. "Only noble motives. But of course he was hardly eager to see you leave for New York to meet me. Right? Refused, in fact, to drive you to the airport when you insisted on going, so you had to take a cab. Right?"

"So what happened?" Mike asks.

"I chose Tony." Doreen laughs. "He was needlessly jealous, but I did what he wanted."

"Right," Tony says. "She humored me. Stupid me. Obsessive me. How could I be so crude as to think David still wanted her?"

"Did he?" Mike asks.

"He pressured me to sleep with him again, but I didn't." Doreen smiles. "It was no big deal."

"No big deal." Tony shakes his head. "I told her I was a very simple man and wanted my life very simple too. I didn't care if I wasn't hip, I didn't care if I sounded uptight, I didn't care if I was a goddamn fossil. Doreen and I had something good going, and I wanted it to last. Christ in heaven, Karen came over one day just after Doreen and I started seeing each other. We hadn't lived together for a year, we hadn't slept together in nearly that long, but I could see Karen wanted me to make it clear that she was more important in my life than Doreen. I could have let them glare at each other, I could have used Karen to make Doreen jealous, but I told her that Doreen and I were in love. Then when she left I told Doreen it was over long since with Karen. And that was that."

"Even so," Mike says, trying now to defend Suzanne, to defend his decision not to ask her not to see Jeff, "it's hard to cut off people like that."

"Listen," Tony responds, "I'm not saying you're the same as me, or that Suzanne and you are the same as Doreen and me. I just didn't want the past to drag us down before we had a chance together. I'm a suspicious bastard. I know myself well enough to see how I used to love to be fought over. That's the way most people are. I had no reason to think Doreen was so different. So I did what I could—I gave her a choice. And promised myself I'd back it up either way. Look at me now." He laughs.

"Well," Mike says, trying to sound determined, "I'm going to get it all straight with Suzanne just as soon as she calls. And she better call soon, or there won't be anything left to get straight." He finishes his beer. "I have to take off. Thanks for the company. Catch you later."

"Good luck," Doreen calls out as Mike heads into the rain.

"Poor bastard," Tony says, closing the front door. "Suzanne doesn't know what the hell she wants."

"She'd be lucky to have Mike," Doreen says. "And you think she'd be sick of Jeff long since."

"It's clear to us, anyway," Tony responds.

Drinking another beer, looking out at the rain, Tony shakes his head, only in part at the thought of what Mike is going to have to work through. He also remembers—all too well—the airport in New York the night Doreen came in from Boston. How much he'd been prepared to lose.

"I chose Tony." Isn't that what Doreen said to Mike? An unfortunate verb, Tony thinks, the suggestion that the outcome had been in doubt. And, "He was needlessly jealous, but I did what he wanted." No, Tony doesn't mind taking the weight, but of course it was unfair of Doreen to imply that that had been the end of it.

Not quite. Not quite. Six months later David came into town, called Doreen when Tony was at work, and met her for coffee. That night, casually, Doreen told Tony she'd seen him.

"How's he doing?" Tony asked, trying to keep his voice even.

"Oh, pretty well," she replied lightly.

"Good job?"

"Yes."

"How's he feeling?"

"Good."

"Glad to hear it."

After a silence of several moments, Tony asked, "Is he living with someone?"

"No. Why?"

"Just wondering," Tony said, "just wondering. How long is he out here?"

"For the summer. He's in a training program. Then they send him back to Boston."

"Does he want to see you again while he's here?"

"I'm sure he does," Doreen said. "After all, we're old friends."

"Feel free," Tony said. "Don't let me stop you."

Doreen eyed him cautiously. "I won't. But thanks anyway."

"Oh," Tony said, "and while you're at it, feel free to get your own place too, if that's what you want."

"For the love of God, Tony," Doreen said, "don't be ridiculous. This isn't the Middle Ages. David and I are just friends."

"I am ridiculous," Tony shouted. "I'm having this conversation. I'm just a fool who happens not to believe this guy's given up on you. You want to see him, fine, that's your choice. Just don't do it around me."

"Tony, come on, why do you have to be so hard on David. He's no threat."

"Hey, I never even met the guy. It's nothing personal. I maybe even owe him something—he's part of what you lived. I'm not trying to deny that or take it away from either of you. But I don't want him in *my* life. That's how I feel. Tell him to get his own old lady."

Doreen was visibly angry for several days, but she didn't move out. Tony assumed that she'd spoken to David again to explain that she wouldn't be seeing him, but refrained from asking her what she'd said. He was afraid to know, really, afraid that she had put the blame on him, compromised him if only in that way.

The summer finally ended. Time passing, David's name came up no more than once in a great while, and each time Tony would accept Doreen's teasing about how jealous he was, how uptight. He accepted it, but he knew better. That summer Tony was searching for a stapler in Doreen's writing desk and saw an envelope tucked under her bankbook. Feeling only a little guilty, he read the letter it contained. From David, of course.

"I can't believe we can't see each other again," Tony read, his blood boiling. "I still love you. He has no right to stop us. He won't even have to know. . . ."

Tony finishes his beer, looks out the window, realizes that the rain has let up. The sky brightens, blue breaks through. Tony never did say anything about the letter to Doreen, unable to bring himself to acknowledge that he'd opened the envelope. And feeling, when his anger subsided, that David's words were a response to Doreen's decision not to see him again. Still, it stuck in his craw.

The phone rings. "Hey, Tony," Mike says. "Sorry I dragged you and Doreen into my crazy love life. I was going nuts, but Suzanne's back now. Everything's fine. We're about to get good and drunk together."

Not about to ask Mike what they had settled between them, or just how much Mike had insisted on knowing about Suzanne's four days, Tony says, "That's good, Mike, real good. Say hi to Suzanne for me."

The Tom in Particular

The cats were pushing for dinner as though they had God on their side, making no allowance for the shift the night before off daylight saving time. The orange tom, having earlier suffered the ignominy of being shooed out for nagging, dropped off the garage roof (from which he could survey most of the human movement in the cottage) onto the redwood fence, sailed to the ground when he reached the gate, and sprinted through the cat door into the kitchen. Arriving at the threshold of the living room with heartfelt urgency, convinced at the very least by his own velocity: surely it was time to eat.

Though the two other cats—the huge tortoiseshell female and her much smaller black-haired mother—spatted obligingly as the tom made his entrance (their strategy being to demonstrate that only hunger pains could drive them to such uncharacteristic squabbling), their mistress was too preoccupied to pay them any mind. She was unpacking, finally, the trunks, bags, and suitcases she'd brought back from her parents' home, the welter of childhood baubles, inherited valuables, and flea-market finds she'd left there for the nearly ten years she'd been on her own.

She'd always insisted that nothing of hers be thrown out, arguing long distance more than once against her mother's resolve to "clean up the children's rooms once and for all." It was not until her parents announced their decision to give up the house for an apartment, however, that she'd gone to fetch what was hers.

Of course she had always kept with her some few treasures. A black cashmere overcoat, once her mother's. Two Mesopotamian spun-gold earrings that tinkled like bells when she wore them. A necklace of black seed pearls given to her grandfather by fishermen on the river Don. And several silver buckles, from a belt of her grandmother's, each engraved with a maiden in profile (right hand cradling a crescent moon, left bearing a garland of lilies).

But at last, now twenty-seven, she finally had all her things again. "Market value four hundred dollars, tops," her husband said from the soft chair in the corner. Newspaper in his lap, shaking himself awake to survey the unpacking.

"Oh, stop it, will you," she said, thinking she'd just as soon be alone. "You don't even know what these things are."

"Artifacts from a previous incarnation? Salvage from Pompeii?"

"Is that supposed to be funny?" she responded sharply. "I don't need to hear it." Just looking at the work ahead made her want quiet and space; she found her husband's voice particularly intrusive. It would help considerably if he—and the cats—just disappeared for a while.

"Sorry. No offense," he said.

Unable to tell from the tone of her husband's voice if he meant it, or if his grin was really apologetic, wondering why she even had to try to figure him out, she glared in his direction. Even this took her far from her thoughts.

"I said I'm sorry. I meant it."

"Okay, okay. Forget it. I'm busy."

Shaking her head, finding none of her husband's tricks amusing, her mind teased by the rush of associations each object summoned up, she walked over to the stereo. Putting on her father's favorite, Stravinsky's *Firebird,* which she'd heard so many times as a child, Pachelbel's Canon in D Major ready to follow, wearing white tights, a black leotard, and black tooled cowboy boots, she began to cull the jumble into three categories.

Clothing

A gray linen schoolgirl's jumper, at least fifteen years old, which still fit her. A sleeveless cotton tennis shirt. A poor-boy sweater with jewel neckline knitted by her sister. Two pairs of straight-leg corduroy pants. "Way too short for my father. Mother got them in a thrift shop."

"What?" her husband asked, busy in the sports page, unable to tell if she was talking to him or to herself.

"Nothing."

Jodhpurs with leather kneepads. A visored riding helmet covered in black velvet. Leather pants. "Ruined," she thought, remembering how years before she'd waded into a saltwater pond when the family's German shepherd had fallen through the ice. And then stood shivering in the cold, watching the dog, memory so short, chasing a cormorant down the beach, while she'd wondered if the pants could be saved. Now, holding them up, inspecting them carefully, she was sure they were finished.

She pressed on. A sky-blue velvet dressing gown with an Elizabethan collar. Two mutton-sleeved bodices: one red silk, the other forest-green taffeta with ivory cuffs and dickey. Anderson tartan Bermuda shorts. A silk Anderson dress-tartan scarf, with bits cut from it. Rosettes for her grandmother's grave.

A skirt of French grosgrain ribbon. A mustard seersucker peasant skirt and blouse. Pleated cream crepe evening pants. An English wool houndstooth jacket. A pair of turn-of-the-century silk ladies' drawers. Her mother's old bathing suit: flowered pleated rayon with full skirt and fitted bodice. Bright pink.

A pinafore with whale spouting. A brick-red Ferragamo knit suit, never worn. A white terrycloth beach jacket. A pencil-cut purple raincoat. A natural raw-silk overcoat, also her mother's.

Chartreuse linen shorts. A Georgian flannel dress with lace collar. An A-line unbleached muslin wraparound skirt, with buttonholes in the shape of dolphins. A velour hat, cabbage green. "I'd never wear something like this, would I?" Her husband, dozing off again, was slow to respond. "Would I?"

"Would you what?"

Material

Black crepe with embroidered silver clouds. Strawberries, lots of them, on a circular flowered patchwork. Organdy and piqué patchwork, all in different whites. Swatches of voile and poplin.

French silk organdy, cloud blue with salmon polka dots. "The color of St. Joseph's Aspirin for Children," she thought. Blue cloth flowers. Satin ribbons. Sequins. A lace butterfly.

Several yards of Chinese linen, small golden horses crossing at full gallop. "It hung over my bed when my room was yellow. I was a horse maiden."

"How old are horse maidens?"

"Are you awake now?"

"More or less."

"I was eleven or twelve. That's horse-maiden age. I had to ride an enormous pinto. Cherokee. He was almost impossible to control. He gave me nightmares. He had a hard mouth."

"What's that?"

"You could rein in hard, but he'd keep on going, biting the horse in front of you. Then that horse would wheel or kick. Cherokee was more like a pony."

"What's wrong with ponies?"

"They're vicious and ornery, cunning, they don't respond easily. Cherokee was full of tricks. He'd rear when you put a foot in the stirrup. Or try to nip the person who was giving you a leg up. When he got too far out of control, my teacher would come over and poke at him with a pointed stick."

"Why did you ride him, then?"

"I had to. It was my teacher's way of making me learn not to give in to a horse. I was always scared of Cherokee, but even so he was a beautiful animal. I loved him."

"Prepubescent maidens turned on by their noble steeds?"

"Very funny."

Usables (and some other things)

Damask curtains. Moss-green linen sheets, soft and worn like flannel. A wicker laundry hamper. "I'm going to paint it white. It should be white." Several silk lamp shades. Red tumbleweed from the Mojave Desert.

Bags of metal shavings (curls of copper and brass). Scissors from Finland. All sorts of biscuit tins, tall and cylindrical, from Fortnum and Mason's or Jackson's of Picadilly. Three Dundee marmalade jars. A picture frame of plaster—painted to look like wood—set on wood, with ailanthus leaves engraved. A pair of finger cymbals for belly dancing. An ornate silver pomegranate.

"What can you do with that?" her husband asked.

"With what?"

"The artificial fruit."

"The pomegranate?"

"If that's what it is. Why does it go with the usables?"

"It's good for storing things in. Like hairpins."

"Oh."

A needlepoint pincushion, filled with sand. Eaton's cards, embossed with her name, for thank-yous her mother had to force her to write. A box of Norell perfumed dusting powder, with puff.

Ernest Thompson Seaton's *Rascal. The Peregrine,* by J. A. Baker. A guide to ferns. *The Art of the Japanese Kite.* Four books on coyotes. And an enormous index, with watercolor illustrations, of North American wild flowers.

Cans of oatmeal, a gift from her mother. Not to be eaten, but to be used instead of soap (packed with a bottle of vinegar for restoring the pH balance to the skin). And from her father, a recording of Donizetti's opera *Betly.*

"Betly's a beautiful girl who spurns her lover."

"Sounds depressingly familiar."

"But she accepts him, finally."

"Then there's hope?"

She paused in her sifting, exhausted. Too much of the past had been opened up, and, with her husband in the room, the present was too well represented. She'd have to take it much slower. In the morning, when he was out of the house. As it was, she'd made it through less than half her things.

Still in the corner in the soft chair, newspaper at his feet, her husband was staring at the disorder as if trying to find something—negative, she thought—to say.

"What's the matter?" she asked.

"Nothing. I was just wondering when you're going to have this mess cleaned up."

"Is that really what's on your mind?"

"No."

"Then what?"

"I've given you lots of things too."

"I know that," she answered, startled to find tears welling in her eyes.

"Well, I forgot. Particularly looking at all your stuff."

"I'd never forget any of your presents."

"Listen. Let's pile everything I've given you in the living room too."

"What? Now?"

Her Husband's Gifts (a partial list)

Three authentic Indian baskets. A treadle sewing machine. One pair of Red Wing Irish Setter work boots. A book of plates of Georgia O'Keeffe's paintings. One down parka, one down sleeping bag. A set of foul-weather gear, including Captains Courageous rain hat. An electric juicer. One rigging knife, one Swiss army knife. An oriole's nest. A wasp's nest. A duck's wing. A set of salmon's teeth. The sound track from *Saturday Night Fever.* "And there's lots more," he said as the pile grew, "not counting the roses for your last birthday. Let me think."

Still not fed, the cats practiced the feline equivalent of Zen meditation: tortoiseshell haunched on the wicker hamper; her black-haired mother curled on the damask; orange tom camped on the chartreuse shorts. The tom in particular despaired that the inventory would ever end.

Broken Wings

Most of the teachers must be retired now; curriculum long since revised and revised again; desks unbolted and replaced by modular furniture; the building itself renovated (interior brick exposed, partitions torn out, skylights installed); students no doubt of a different breed altogether. In the mid-fifties, however, Sheldon gave no sign of a capacity for change, was as it had been for generations of students, countless older brothers and sisters. Because Sheldon was the smallest of the city's six grammar schools, no more than twenty-five students in each class, nearly all the eighth-grade boys were needed to field the "varsity" teams. Even Jack Hurley—six-three, one hundred and thirty pounds, body phenomenally beyond his control—generally got to walk around the halls in uniform on game days. Most of the eighth-grade girls were cheerleaders or majorettes. So much of the class in the event itself, the rooting section was usually almost empty.

Dino was never a team captain—too subversive—but he was always a leader. Not because, at thirteen, he appeared to care much, but because even overweight he was far and away the best athlete. He'd come down court in basketball, throw up a left-handed hook just to see what happened, and, laughing, watch it go in. Or he'd point to right field in a baseball game, like Babe Ruth calling his shot, and then punch the ball over the first baseman's head. No other player even toyed with the possibility of placing the ball. But under all his flab, though he could never shinny a rope in gym class, Dino had tremendous coordination.

He also knew sports up and down. Batting averages, team standings, records for all categories. He had a short-wave radio and followed the various Boston teams even when they were on the road, staying up past midnight to hear the final scores. Then showing up at school at 7:15 to shoot hoops, doing a frenzied play-by-play of his moves à la Johnny Most, the Celtics' crazily partisan announcer.

It was not only out of respect for athletic ability that Dino's friends never criticized him for being such an incredible brownnoser. He was so excessive, and had started so late (abruptly, after summer vacation, at the beginning of eighth grade), that they had trouble believing the teachers went for it. Dino actually brought apples for Mrs. White. Waved his arms like a mad conductor when she entered the classroom, presumably signaling for silence, but in fact compounding the chaos. He had to be kidding, but he even stayed after school to clean her blackboards and carry her things downstairs. Because grades were given for both performance and attitude, his labors were doubly rewarded.

Or perhaps his friends never thought the less of Dino because, no matter what he did to get all A's, they believed that the brownnosing was some kind of game for him, something he'd one day reveal his distance from, laughing. Even as he scored most of the points in a basketball game, for instance, he'd be grinning at the coach, Mr. Conroy, for taking it so seriously. Shaking his head at the ineptness of the boy guarding him. Applauding the cheerleaders as they cheered him, like Khrushchev after a speech to the Presidium. Jack Hurley, on the bench all but thirty seconds of the game, would watch Dino, way past envy to admiration. Dino was everything, Jack thought, that he'd never be: in control of himself, in control of the situation, so free of what was around him that he could laugh. Jack's father, himself six-seven, often told Jack that he'd fill out, that he'd be a fine athlete someday. But Jack knew he'd never be like Dino. No one would.

Dino, however, was serious about wanting the Cummings Award, given each year to the student with the highest grade point in the graduating (eighth-grade) class. His brother had won it several years before, and Dino was under great pressure from his family to do the same. Knowing there were brighter students, Dino tried whatever might work, even leading the chorus, since it too was graded. Yet even as he started off the school song at assemblies, booming away, he winked at his friends to show them how foolish it all was.

Sheldon, O Sheldon, we will never leave you,
Though our paths lead even o'er the sea.
You guide our purposes, you light our memories,
Through thick and thin, no matter where we may be.

Like Joey Conn, Mike MacFarlane, and the others, Jack Hurley always studied Dino's lips to see if he was singing the revised lyrics he'd come up with one day.

Sheldon, down Sheldon, we don't want to see you,
That's why we're going far o'er the sea.
You have no purpose, you blight our memories.
Take our advice and please let us be.

The danger was that they'd break out laughing, though Dino could always control himself, grinning but just composed enough. Miss Malone, in fact, had hauled Jack Hurley and some of Dino's other friends down to her office after school to get them to tell her what was so funny. They missed basketball practice for a week but wouldn't betray him.

By Christmas that year in eighth grade, however, Dino realized that Janet Burroughs, loathed by the class for her years of humorless ass-kissing, was going to beat him out. She'd received an A in homemaking, Dino a B-plus in shop. Mr. Michaelson really liked him, but Dino had almost no mechanical aptitude. As it was, the grade was a gift. If Dino was disappointed he didn't let on, but after vacation he stopped brownnosing the teachers as abruptly as he'd begun, leaving them high and dry. Mrs. White asked several students if Dino was feeling all right.

Disappointments aside, eighth grade was definitely the place to be. All the marshalls were eighth-graders (red armband on left biceps), which meant extra time to walk the corridors between classes. Projector operators and pedestrian-crosswalk supervisors were also eighth-graders. More free time, missed classes. In addition, the teachers tended to be loose with the oldest students. They'd seen most of them around, after all, for eight years. If by now they couldn't trust them, didn't like them, what pleasure was there in the vocation? Sentimentality—and a desire for peace—obscured many a sin. Only Miss Malone never relented, poured it on, in fact, determined that her students, excelling in high school, would be living testimonials to her pedagogy. Yet even her assignments to memorize long passages from *Evangeline* ("This is the forest primeval. The murmuring pines and the hemlocks . . .") failed to dampen the eighth-graders' spirits. They were, for the moment, on top.

Weekdays between eight-twenty and three, Sheldon was the world, the morning Lord's Prayer and Pledge of Allegiance reinforcing a sense of order and continuity. Yet though the students were generally no more than fourteen when they graduated, of course they were long since part of the larger community. Betty Duffy's mother drank heavily and beat her. Ned Farley's parents had divorced; he lived with his grandparents. Joey Cohn was seeing a psychiatrist four times a week, and avoided going right home after school because his mother had a lover. Jack Fink's house burned down. Susie Goldstein's parents went bankrupt. Tommy Goode was picked up for shoplifting and then for stealing bicycles. Elaine Simms was pregnant and had to leave school; slightly retarded, she was nearly sixteen. Jerry Venucci's father, allegedly a Mafioso, was in prison. Mike MacFarlane had already been in reform school; he liked to take off his jacket and shirt on bitterly cold days, rub snow on his chest, and brandish an enormous switchblade. Mr. Alden, Sheldon's principal, had acquired an arsenal of weapons he'd confiscated from Mike.

Though in these terms Dino had no special claim to fame, his father had died the summer before. He went slowly and was home most of the time, ever more gaunt, skin jaundiced, whites of his eyes yellow.

Dino's friends were sorry, of course, but after the funeral he quickly seemed himself. Because his mother worked late, Dino now had tremendous freedom. The way his friends saw it, it was just like Dino to have such good fortune. He was exempt, somehow, from the rules that bound them. Just as he never practiced but excelled at sports, so he was the only one who could mention reform school to Mike MacFarlane without getting beaten up. Dino would ask Mike if, being so tough, he could eat nails, if they'd taught him that while he was locked up. To the amazement of the other boys, Mike loved it. And Dino would ask Joey Cohn if his psychiatrist was coming to see some Sheldon basketball games, or if Joey had told him about Dino's hook shot. No one was supposed to know about the psychiatrist, but Joey would laugh. Even the class president, Stevie Crane, handsome in the obligatory way—no pimples, blond hair, a smile that offended no one—understood that Dino was far beyond him.

Not long after Christmas that year, the eighth grade learned that it was to put on the next play, for Washington's Birthday. As usual, the whole school and interested parents would attend. The skits Mrs. White devised had little that seemed original, even to the eighth-graders. *Moments in Our Country's History,* she called the mélange. Washington chopping down the cherry tree, of course. Lincoln delivering the Gettysburg Address. Paul Revere making his ride. Squanto helping the Pilgrims. Pocahontas saving John Smith. Several other skits, various musical interludes, and a finale in which all twenty-five eighth-graders would sing "America the Beautiful" and "God Bless America." The assembly would end, as all Sheldon assemblies ended, with everyone rising to join in "Sheldon, O Sheldon."

Dino was George Washington and also controlled the curtain, a position of some responsibility. The performance began as usual, each grade filing in, parents seated at the rear of the auditorium, the six-piece orchestra painfully emitting an overture of patriotic melodies. After he opened the curtain, Dino—who never had stage fright—stepped to the lights in his wig and knickers and could not tell a lie. Jerry Venucci, playing to a group of his father's "business associates" in the audience, rode a broomstick to Lexington and Concord. Betty Duffy, as Betsy Ross, sewed stars on America's first flag. Janet Burroughs sang a solo version of "This Is My Country" and then encored with "Oklahoma!" Dino closed the curtain after her second bow. End of Act One.

When, after an intermission of several minutes, he opened it again, Ned Farley, in blackface, sang "Old Man River." Joey Cohn then freed the slaves. Tommy Goode showed the Pilgrims how to plant fish under the cornseed. Susie Goldstein saved John Smith. Janet Burroughs had protested to Mrs. White that Susie and Tommy should be in Act One, but Mrs. White had informed her, coolly, that these were only "vignettes," that a certain liberty could be taken with the "traditional unities."

Susie Goldstein, in any case, had just finished when Dino did something very strange. He closed the curtain. Though there had been perfunctory applause for Susie, the audience, now concluding that the play was over, began to clap more vigorously. There was more than a little surprise on the part of students and teachers watching, however, because traditionally—always, that is to say—a production number with the whole class was the finale. Backstage, in fact, the eighth-graders had been waiting to gather, but as the applause grew they stood confused. Mrs. White jumped up from her seat in the front row, her fixed smile gone now, but it was, suddenly, too late. Assembly apparently finished, the audience rose and began to sing "Sheldon, O Sheldon."

"I blew it," Dino shouted from behind the curtain as he heard them begin, though to that moment his error—and surely it was an error—could have been reversed. His voice was probably not heard by the audience, their lungs full, but it triggered a strong response in his classmates. Realizing that precedent had been broken, anything seemed possible, anything at all, and they began to run back and forth across the stage. A set toppled. Betty Duffy screamed. Mike MacFarlane saw a bass drum and began to beat it, hard. Susie Goldstein started crying. Jack Hurley, who had tripped, causing the set to fall, stood rooted to the spot, afraid to lose control again by setting himself in motion.

Meanwhile, Mr. Alden was standing in front of the audience, as he always did after a performance, trying to thank "Mrs. White and our eighth-graders for their wonderful and edifying presentation," but he hurried his remarks to conclusion as the noise behind him increased. Peeking through the curtain, Dino saw him heading backstage looking very angry. Mr. Alden had an enormous nose, which none of the students were supposed to notice, much less mention. "It's the Beak," Dino shouted, and eighth-graders poured out the fire doors.

Censure of the class continued to and through graduation. Teachers repeatedly told each other that they'd never seen anything like it. Miss Malone made her classes sit in silence for a week and then gave them test after test. Mrs. White took a month of sick leave. No one received the Cummings Award, though Janet Burroughs's parents protested. There were no predictions of great things for the class. And, strangely, no one ever asked Dino why he'd closed the curtain. It was assumed that he'd of course just lost his head in the excitement of the performance. But on the other hand, his friends thought, Dino was always in control. No one said anything about it.

Finally the eighth-graders graduated and, after summer vacation, started at the bottom again at high school. That fall Dino played basketball but quit well before the season ended. The coach was too serious, he said, and he was feeling tremendous pressure from his mother about grades. His brother had just started Cornell, but Dino was doing no better than B work in most of his classes. Worse, he was having real trouble with Latin.

A tiny man near retirement age, who wore heavy wool suits in all seasons, Mr. Crowley was devoted to Latin and expected much from his students. Each week he assigned a tremendous list of words to be memorized. Up late listening to basketball and football games, Dino soon fell behind. He cheated on one test, using a trot in his lap, but the tension was getting to him. He spent most of his time with Jack Hurley, Joey Cohn, Tommy Goode, Mike MacFarlane, and the others from Sheldon, making few attempts to get to know his new classmates. Though he bantered as always, he was also occasionally moody, surprising his friends.

In fact, Dino had good reason to feel uneasy. Afraid to show his mother his first-semester grades, he'd stolen a blank report card from the principal's office, filled in false grades—A's—given his mother the phony card to sign, and then forged his mother's name on the real one. It had worked, but Dino was under great stress.

The second semester of first-year Latin, Mr. Crowley always had each student read aloud from the text, *Caesar's Commentaries.* A methodical soul, he invariably began with the row of students on his far right, moved up it, then down the next, and so on, quietly asking each successive student to "read the Latin." Dino was lucky: his seat was on Mr. Crowley's far left, and he had plenty of time to prepare the pages from which he'd have to read and translate. But he found it hard to make himself concentrate, kept falling further behind on the list of words.

He covered his nervousness well most of the time, still always joking with his friends, talking like Johnny Most, doing imitations of Mr. Crowley and the other teachers. But then one day he came to school with a brown paper lunch bag. "I've got a Drano sandwich," he told his friends. They cracked up, though in fact they didn't know what to make of it. Dino was incredible, they all said, really incredible. The next day he appeared again with a lunch bag. Another Drano sandwich, he told them. But fresh bread.

This continued each day for the next week, and, except for laughing each time, none of his friends thought much about it. They couldn't figure out what Dino was up to, but he'd show them when he was ready. They could trust him for that. Mr. Crowley, meanwhile, like the *Titanic*'s iceberg, had reached Dino's row. There were now three students between Dino and Mr. Crowley. The first had a rough time and consumed nearly the whole period in a futile attempt to translate ten lines. Mr. Crowley was deeply disappointed.

The next day Dino again brought a lunch bag and mentioned the Drano sandwich. This time, however, he announced that he was going to eat it. Not then, but soon. His friends really laughed. A typical Dino move. How would he do it?

In Latin class Mr. Crowley called on one of the two students between him and Dino, listened carefully to the reading and translation, and then digressed for twenty minutes to talk about what England had been like in Caesar's day. This presentation was hardly spur-of-the-moment. Mr. Crowley had about thirty short lectures typed up and delivered one from time to time as the school year progressed. This day, in any case, he spoke until the bell rang and then dismissed the class.

The next morning Dino told his friends that he'd eat the Drano sandwich that afternoon, in Latin class. Again they laughed. How would he carry it off? Not only were they unable to envision what Dino had in mind, but also, during the previous week, they'd become accustomed both to the word "Drano" and the apparent oxymoron "Drano sandwich." They were certain, of course, that something would happen. As indeed it did. When the class filed in, the student in front of Dino was absent. After waiting to make sure, Dino reached for his lunch bag, opened the wax paper, took the sandwich in his hands, and stuffed it into his mouth. Mr. Crowley was just lifting his eyes from the plan book to ask Dino to "read the Latin."

"I'm dying, I'm dying," Dino bellowed, and toppled to the floor. "I'm burning to death. Help me." Poor Mr. Crowley. Nothing like this had ever happened before. He ran to the hall, pulled the fire alarm, and, one hand on his heart, the other on the banister, he rushed downstairs to get the nurse.

Carried out on a stretcher, his stomach pumped, Dino was taken by ambulance to the hospital. Though he was there recuperating for several weeks, he suffered only some burns in his mouth and throat. Restricted to a liquid diet, he drank countless chocolate milkshakes. In time, he returned to school and to Latin class. Saddened each day he saw Dino, Mr. Crowley always made a point of speaking to him gently, asking him when his turn came if he could "read the Latin."

The afternoon Dino ate the Drano sandwich the story was all over the high school, and most students simply thought he was crazy. Dino's friends, however, were devastated. They visited him in the hospital but never found the words to ask him why he'd done it.

There were several other effects of Dino's Drano sandwich. At the least, the boys from Sheldon remained a close group throughout high school, never really mixing with the larger student body. And Dino's friends, each in a different way, dealt individually with what he'd done. Mike MacFarlane broke the nose of an upperclassman who laughed at Dino in the corridor one day, and went back to reform school for six months. Joey Cohn spent hours with his psychiatrist trying to figure out why Dino had done it, what it meant. And Jack Hurley, by the end of freshman year six-five and one hundred and fifty pounds, started shooting hoops each day for hours, determined to make the junior varsity team sophomore year. For Dino.

Years later, scattered around the country, Dino's friends occasionally wondered what had happened to him. Remembering his Johnny Most impersonations and how much he'd loved sports, they hoped he'd become an announcer. So much, still, did they respect what he'd been that none would have been surprised to see him on TV doing play-by-play for "Monday Night Football."

Mike MacFarlane, mirabile dictu, was now a cop, Joey Cohn a professor of comparative literature, Jerry Venucci a doctor, Stevie Crane a hair stylist. Who would have guessed? Jack Hurley had played college basketball, toyed with turning pro, but gone into law instead. Now he had a good practice, was happily married, and had a son of his own. Once, only once, at a party, everyone drunk and reminiscing about school days, Jack recounted the story of Dino and the Drano sandwich. Dismayed, in the telling, and feeling he'd let Dino down, when several of his friends began to laugh.

Some Savage Present

My parents always had a dog. A Great Dane, before the children were born, when they lived in the country. By the time I was compos mentis we had Jake, a German shepherd. As soon as I was old enough, I took him out each morning before school as part of my household chores. We had several large parks nearby; there was plenty of room for him to run. When it snowed, he'd get his exercise chasing my sled down the hill, nipping at the runners.

My mother, who often walked five or six miles a day on her errands, generally took Jake with her. Often I saw her come into view at the far end of the street, carrying her packages but still striding strongly, Jake somewhat behind, tongue hanging.

Though well trained, Jake lost some of the circulation to his brain and began to be a menace, attacking the postman and delivery boys, and finally had to be put to sleep. We immediately got another shepherd, a pup, who had a fine pedigree but seemed to lack some essential. Despite long sessions at obedience school, Slouch (my younger sister named him) never really grasped the basic commands. In frustration the instructor would pull him around on a short leash with a choke collar, but always Slouch responded by trying to lick the man's face. We felt embarrassed standing there in the converted garage as the other dog owners watched, but it was impossible not to love Slouch.

Though he never quite got it all together, Slouch was without malice and, I hope, felt no pain. He was, however, dominated by our cat Maestro, who each afternoon would egg Slouch into whining for dinner long before there was any possibility they'd be fed—they ate from the same bowl—and would then watch, very calmly, as Slouch was punished. Maestro also liked to run along when Slouch was walked on leash, as if to remind him of his lack of freedom. Though he never matured, Slouch aged and finally died, but by then I was off at college. I see him best in a photo taken during my childhood. My little sister, about four or five, dressed in rubber boots, heavy coat, scarf, and coonskin cap, is kissing Slouch on the head, inadvertently scrunching his eyes with her mittened hands as she does so.

For years after I left home I had little to do with the canine world, except when I came down in some dog shit after making a dazzling catch in touch football, or when I saw yet another longhair with a dog—red bandanna for a collar—I suspected would soon be abandoned. I do remember that a couple I knew had two Great Danes, intelligent, aloof, beautifully trained, that I would gladly have accepted as my own.

I again lived around dogs when I worked on a ranch. There the Border collies were more useful than a dozen horsemen, a marvel to watch as they circled behind cows or sheep to bunch them up. Though the dogs were born for this work, it was easy to pity them. Sleeping through endless days chained next to their fifty-five-gallon-drum houses, the dogs were there to handle the stock. The rancher loved them but had no time for pets. When he didn't need them, which was most of the time, they waited, watching carefully each time he passed for some sign that they were about to be released.

I recount all this to preface what follows, lest I seem a born dog-hater. One can apparently distinguish between dog people and cat people, but I was raised with both, loved both. And while I now have cats, I tend to think of them as my wife's (except when a neighborhood boy throws a firecracker their way on the Fourth of July). I'd have a dog now, I'm sure, were cities not such cruel places for them.

If, in any case, what I've told you were all I knew about dogs, or if I'd never returned to the city, we could stop here. My troubles began when I moved next door to a Canadian man perhaps fifty years old. A garrulous and interesting soul, he'd traveled much of his life. Now, living simply, he told wonderful tales about his wanderings and had a white beard that made him appear older than he was. He also owned three dogs, to which he was obviously devoted. In time, I learned that he trained dogs professionally. He seemed to know what he was doing, and I was particularly impressed by his quiet firmness. If he wanted to teach a dog to be quiet, for instance, he simply tapped it on the nose each time it barked. No big deal, but it worked.

As I got to know him better, I saw that he was a troubled man, lonely and an alcoholic. Sometimes he'd have eight or ten dogs in his apartment, being paid to train or board them, but he'd pass out, and the dogs, needing exercise, would bark and fight. More than once I asked him to keep them quiet. Each time he invited me in for a drink to make amends, promising that it would never happen again. But nothing changed. Soon he and I were arguing bitterly.

There were several impediments to an easy solution. To begin with, he had a way of suggesting that I was simply uptight, that if I looked more closely I might see that he was a latter-day Saint Francis of Assisi. Indeed, this gave me pause, not because his flaws weren't all too obvious, but because I had no desire to be cast in the role of the heavy. Who would? Second, I couldn't hit him because he was too old: I'd feel bad. And, finally, he was an illegal alien, so I was loath to call the police to enforce the health ordinance regulating the number of dogs in a residence.

My anger only increased when I realized that he knew I wouldn't hit him or call the authorities. The wily bastard was sure, in fact, that I'd shut up or move. He had me. I began looking for a new place but found immediately that there was nothing comparable to mine. I checked the paper each day, went to bulletin boards, called friends, searched for anything reasonable. But how was I going to replace cheap rent, the beautiful blood roses, my view of the hills and rising moon, the lovely porch room next to the plum tree? I returned each day from my hunt to see him sitting on his door stoop. Grinning.

I began to joke to friends about throttling him to death, and, though they considered my humor in bad taste, I knew I had cause. He'd added insult to injury by augmenting his canine population with a pack of teenagers who were crashing with him.

They, needless to say, considered him a pure spirit. Like him, however, they were too drunk or drugged to wake when fire broke out in his room. Two senior citizens, neighbors who had also complained about the dogs, called the fire department and then went in through the smoke to rouse the teenagers and drag him out. Man and dog alike were saved. Life continued as before.

In desperation I rented a small cottage that was overpriced and already furnished (nothing could be changed) right out of the Sears catalog. My wife thought I was crazy to take it but bit her tongue when I said that if we didn't move right then I'd kill him. There was worse news, however. My new landlady lived next door. She had two Labradors, and her three children—collective IQ perhaps 93—delighted in taunting the Japanese woman in the house behind us whenever she complained about the dog excrement and the flies. "Clean it up, clean it up, clean it up, use your hands, use your hands," the children would chant.

We finally found another cottage to rent, and when the landlord put it up for sale we bought it. My buyer's remorse is another sorry saga, but in fact we were soon more comfortable, painting the inside, putting in a large garden, building some fences. The only hitch was that there were almost as many dogs as people in the neighborhood. This may sound hyperbolic, but there was in fact a dog for almost every household, and some families had several. Further, many of the lots had been subdivided, so that there were perhaps twenty-five dogs within a three-hundred-foot radius of my new home.

I don't know just what I expected when I began to speak to my neighbors about their dogs. Did I have some vision of community? Did I anticipate reasoned discourse, a meeting of the minds? Could I have even dreamed of compromise? Whatever, I was quickly disabused. There had recently been a rash of robberies, and then a rapist had started to work the area. Even people who loathed dogs now kept one stationed in the yard.

My first attempt at discussing the problem was with an aged neighbor who lived around the corner. She thought me mad to begin with, since I didn't even live on her street. This conviction persisted though I pointed out that our homes were less than a hundred feet apart, that in addition the prevailing wind carried her dog's barking right through my closed windows. We spoke at some length, but it finally dawned on me that she wanted the dog to bark, felt safer when it did. I then asked, didn't she really want it to bark only when someone set foot on her property? Did she actually want to scare off the neighbor who started his car each morning to go to work? Something in this question seemed perverse to her: she snorted in disgust, told me I was wasting her time, and slammed the door in my face. I came back to my cottage, steaming, and slammed my door.

My next encounter was with a professor who lived across the street with a French poodle. Expecting the worst now, I began to explain to him what I hoped he would do, and, to my utter amazement, he immediately apologized, saying that he would keep the dog inside and arrange for it to be walked when he was gone. I couldn't believe my ears, was positively inarticulate in my thanks. And I never really heard his poodle again, except when I occasionally passed his door and discerned a muffled woofing that might have been the dog.

Thus inspired, several days later I approached the house next to his, greeted by a woman in her thirties. She had an air of hard-earned independence, the aura of living without a man and liking it, possibly also radical sympathies. No matter, I thought. Sex preferences weren't the question, or politics. I'd just tell it like it was.

Once again I began my explanation of my mission, but she cut me off to say, impatiently, that her dog's barking didn't bother *her*. Since this remark seemed profoundly irrelevant to all I'd just so earnestly set forth, I wrestled with a response. It did of course follow in some obscure way, if only because she'd said it, but I was hampered by the thought I'd given to my argument. Trying to make my presentation as logical as possible, each small step leading inevitably to the next, moving finally to the inescapable conclusion that the dog would have to be stopped from barking.

I needn't have bothered. "My dog's an Irish setter," she added, before I could speak.

"I know that," I managed to respond, confused by what seemed to me another, and stranger, non sequitur. "But . . ."

"Just imagine," she said, interrupting me, "that when you hear it barking you're in Ireland."

"You vicious bitch," I said to myself, unwilling to say it to her since I still hoped to somehow salvage the encounter. And get her dog to stop barking. Fond hope! She was staring at me in triumph. I decided, therefore, to settle for satisfaction.

"And when I hear the Doberman down the street," I said, "should I think of Vienna, the Rhine, and Goethe, or should I see Nazi storm troopers and smoke from the death camps?"

"Fuck you," she replied. I'd won the battle but, of course, had lost the war.

It took me a number of weeks to recover from this exchange, but I finally decided to deal with my immediate neighbors, who only recently had acquired a beautiful springer spaniel pup. Both adults worked all day and left the dog out in the back yard. Behind a fence, hearing people and dogs pass, the pup barked constantly. Further, the garbage men came by each Monday and Thursday morning—at seven. Particularly outraged by the sound of trash cans being banged around and the whine of the truck's compressor, the pup began barking as soon as he heard the garbage men down the street, and kept up a frenzy of high yelps until they passed on to another neighborhood.

Since my last face-to-face confrontation had been so fruitless, I plotted a new strategy and left a typewritten note on my neighbors' door. "I'm sorry to distrub you with this," I wrote, "but I have to complain about your dog's barking. While I happen to like dogs . . ." Reading it over, I thought I'd done pretty well, especially with the phrase "reciprocal consideration."

Perhaps three days later I heard a knock on my front door. The whole family was out there—two parents, one son, and the pup.

"We want to introduce ourselves," Papa said, "to show you we're good people. As you can see, the dog is just a puppy."

I held my head to keep it from exploding. "I never doubted that you are good people," I said, trying to choose my words carefully. "You have a nice puppy and seem like a nice family. But for the love of God, please stop it from barking all day long, day after day." Oops! I'd made a mistake with that last line.

"I can't believe Rowley barks 'all day,' " Mama said.

"Madam," I answered, with, I'm afraid, a voice that was more than a little snide, "what possible benefit could there be to disparaging your Rowley?"

"I just can't believe it," she said, meaning, of course, that she just couldn't believe *me.* "My son tells me the dog is very quiet."

I'd had it. The kid was inside every afternoon making out with his girl friend. He wouldn't notice Nagasaki. So that made me a liar. Screw it!

"Ask the dog," I finally said. "It looks like an honest dog. Or should I run a tape while your dog barks and then play it back for you at full volume around three in the morning?"

But Mama wasn't listening. Off they went, not a word of farewell.

I called the police as soon as they crossed my property line, got the emergency service by mistake, and had to call in again. My conversation on this pressing matter was recorded. Between beeps, I gathered from the officer that there was a nuisance statute on the books which covered barking. Following his suggestion, I called the pound and learned of a process that began with delivery of a notice of complaint and, theoretically, progressed to the impoundment of the animal if I persisted. Elated, I asked them to deliver the initial notice. Almost immediately the puppy barked less, but always, still, when the garbage men appeared. I also observed that the family avoided me whenever our paths threatened to cross.

The pound had helped, apparently, but I sensed that only the easily intimidated would respond so quickly. Further, one of the dogcatchers told me that no one had ever successfully removed a dog by following the complaint process. About all the pound really did was deliver notices. Then one day I was sitting outside and saw several women in uniform dragging a dog out from under a car. It turned out that they were from the pound and were enforcing the leash law.

"Don't do that," I said. "This dog just sits on the curb waiting for its mistress to come home from work. Of all the dogs to pick! You only caught it because it's well trained and gentle. I ought to know. I'm at war with people who have dogs that are out of control, but please don't take this one."

The two women looked at me as if I threatened bodily harm and moved furtively toward the two-way radio. All right, I thought. To hell with them. To hell with the pound.

Several days later I heard a new bark at around six-thirty in the morning. It was very close, and, still in bed, eyes closed, I located it two houses over. Trying to go back to sleep, failing, I put on my robe and slippers. When I knocked on the door a young woman, baby on hip, answered.

"Sorry to bother you," I began, and once more delivered my appeal. This time, however, I invoked Kant's categorical imperative, at the same time modulating my voice to a fine secure tone. Indeed, I was proud of how gently I was speaking, a pure lullaby of explanation and logic. I concluded by pleading for consideration.

"I'll tell my husband," she said, which seemed a rather strange response. That is, apparently disclaiming any personal responsibility. But it was a beginning. I'd seen worse. "Thank you very much," I said, and departed.

I was away in the country for several weeks—heard some coyotes but no dogs, praise the Lord—but the night I returned their animal howled frantically for more than an hour. Though it was late, I went over to their house and knocked on the door.

"You may remember me," I said, risking understatement, when the same young woman appeared. "I've come to ask you to do something about the barking. I have to work early in the morning. I hope you don't think it too difficult to show some consideration for your neighbors."

Suddenly she burst into tears. "I hate the dog," she sobbed. "It belongs to my husband. I told him what you said. I want him to get rid of the dog."

"I'm sorry," I muttered. "I don't mean to cause you any trouble. I don't think you have to get rid of the dog. Just train it—that's not hard—or keep it inside. Anyway, please tell your husband I came by. Sorry."

Several nights later the dog again barked and howled for more than an hour. I was trying to do my taxes and was going insane. Again I walked over to their house. This time the husband came to the door. I had just started to say something when he interrupted me.

"Hey, you're the asshole who hassled my wife."

"Me?"

"Aren't you the one who came around before?"

"Yes, but to ask that the dog be kept quiet."

"You had no right to talk to my wife."

"For Christ's sake," I said. "How in the name of all that's holy would I know that I'm not supposed to talk to your wife? She answered the door, looked healthy enough, and, for all I knew, owned the dog. All I asked her to do was stop the dog from barking. If the dog was quiet I'd have never come over the first time."

"Listen," he said somewhat menacingly, and I now noticed that he was about six-foot-four, 250 pounds, ponytail down to his shoulders, gold stud in his left ear. Cut the sleeves of his denim jacket, show him how to French kiss his buddies, and you'd have a Hell's Angel. I grinned inadvertently when the thought sprang into my mind that he also looked like Lumpjaw in *Bongo the Bear*. But he was speaking, and I listened. "You want to talk about the dog you talk to me. I don't want you over here with my wife."

I must have been crazy, but I was well past the point of no return. "Look, I wasn't *with* your wife, I asked her to stop the dog from barking. I didn't want to talk to her, and I don't really want to talk to you. In fact, you won't see me again. This time I'll call the police."

"What do you mean 'call the police,' " he said, his voice suddenly more moderate. "What kind of shit is that?"

"Look," I said, sensing that I'd found his weak spot. "Your dog is a cannon, and you're firing it at me. Keep it inside, take it with you, have someone walk it, but if you don't shut it up I'll call the police."

"But I can't keep it inside," he replied, "that's not fair to the dog."

My mind boggled. "Not fair to the dog? What about your neighbors?"

"Asshole," he said as I stalked off.

I stormed back to my cottage, certain that nothing would improve and that I might get my head knocked up my nethers if I wasn't careful.

"How'd it go?" my wife asked.

"Got 'em on the run," I muttered, closing the door to my study to continue work on just how much I owed Uncle Sam.

Weeks passed, but nothing changed. I'd thought that Lumpjaw was an escaped convict and would quiet the dog to stop me from calling the police, but apparently I was wrong. Meanwhile, tired of bureaucracies and, at best, slow gains, I thought of going beyond the law. I couldn't really stomach the idea of murdering the animal, however, and if my wife—a walking chapter of the SPCA—even caught me thinking about it she'd nail my ears to the wall. I did consider dognapping, I admit. If I could just lure Lumpjaw's pride and joy out to my car with some prime beef, I could drive across the Bay to San Francisco and release it. There was no way in the world a quadruped could get back over. And I'd be doing it a favor, since nothing could be worse than being locked up all day.

I also thought of having my friend Mad Dog pay a courtesy call on Lumpjaw to reason with him—with his lead pipe. But much as this made me smile, I was afraid the whole business might escalate out of control. The cats. My house. Lumpjaw clearly thought he was some kind of cowboy, might even have a gun. No, there had to be a better way.

As the garbage men were working the street one morning, dogs howling, it occurred to me that Lumpjaw was a tenant. I'd find the owner, make him take care of the problem. His property, after all. His profit. His responsibility.

I called the tax office, gave them the address, and asked for the owner's name. I was put on hold, and after about ten minutes a woman came on to explain that because of Proposition 13 and the budget cuts, the department was understaffed.

"And," I said.

"There's no one here who can go look up your information."

"What are *you* doing?"

"Uh-uh. Can't touch it. Not my job."

"Not your job?" I said.

"Right."

"How far are the files?"

"From where?"

"From where you are right now."

"Other side of the room."

"How big is the room?"

"Not that big."

"Can I tell you something?" I said. I was losing control.

"What?"

"Forget it, just forget it. Let me talk to your supervisor."

"She's busy right now."

"What's her name?"

"All right, hold on."

After another ten-minute wait, message units clicking off steadily, the supervisor came on the line.

"Can I help you?"

Her voice sounded both competent and polite, so I began again. "Sorry to bother you. I know you're short-handed, but I didn't vote for Jarvis-Gann, and I'm in deep trouble. Can you help me?"

She could and did, and that same day I was knocking on Michael Murphy's front door. It turned out that he lived in the duplex in front of Lumpjaw's cottage. Murphy answered and immediately invited me in, though it was clear he hadn't listened to what I said I was after. He just wanted company, any company: at eighty, his days were slow. I told him about the barking dog, but he said that he'd never heard it. Too deaf. I assured him that it did bark and asked if he'd take care of it.

"What do you want me to do?" he said.

"I think you should get the tenant to keep the dog inside, have it trained, or get it walked during the day so it calms down."

"I can't do that."

"Why not?"

"Too old."

"Are you too old to collect his rent check every month?" I asked, utterly exasperated.

"I'll see," was all he'd say, and he ushered me to the door. I must have really aggravated him: he was so lonely that he'd have talked the ear off the neighborhood rapist.

"You better," I shouted to make sure he heard me. "Otherwise, I'm taking you and your tenant to court."

I was manifestly insane by this time, but not without allies, my fellow sufferers. Several of my neighbors had been over to see Lumpjaw. No visible help. When one returned to complain late one night, Lumpjaw's wife came to the door, chased him around the corner to his place, and then stood on the curb screaming at him: "How can I keep the dog inside? Do you want it to shit in the house? You're crazy, crazy, crazy."

At this point my wife finally heard the dog barking. For months, since we left the apartment when the Canadian drove me wild, she'd looked at me as though I was overreacting. But suddenly she reached her limit and got into the fray. She was wild when she returned from Lumpjaw's. "The dog is being mistreated," she said. "I'm going to notify the Humane Society. No, I can't do that. They'll just take the dog away and, when nobody claims it, they'll destroy it. I'll have to talk to the owner."

I was opposed to her doing this, and we argued for hours. My fellow sufferers and I had already contacted the police and, finally, filed a criminal complaint against both Lumpjaw and his landlord. Now, having gone through so much, I no longer just wanted the dog to stop barking. I wanted a victory.

There was no way to stop my wife, of course. When she finally found them home she was there an hour, and returned with the key to their cottage.

"What's that for?" I asked.

"If Saber barks I'm supposed to put him inside."

"Saber?"

"The dog."

"For Christ's sake," I said, "who wants to know its name? Why do you have to meddle in this now?"

"Take it easy. They're not such bad people. He's working two jobs, and she has the baby. The rent's too high. He doesn't want trouble with the neighbors, he really doesn't."

"What about last night when the dog barked for an hour?"

"They were out. He forgot to bring Saber in. He told me that when he remembered they were already in San Francisco."

"Why doesn't he just get rid of the damn thing?"

" He and Saber love each other. You should have seen them playing."

"Wonderful." The truth was that I couldn't afford to hear it. How could Lumpjaw warrant my sympathy now? I was taking him to court. Damn my wife!

Several days later he left a note on my windshield. "I've given my dog away," it said. "Fuck you."

"Fuck you too," I thought, called my fellow plaintiffs, and broke open a bottle of schnapps. We'd won. Loath to go home, I lingered over the bottle with them.

"He got rid of Saber," my wife said as I walked in the door.

"Right."

"I hope you're satisfied. He gave Saber to the Humane Society. They'll just put him to sleep."

"Someone will take him," I answered, without much conviction.

"I hope you're satisfied," she said again.

The living room couch wasn't that uncomfortable, but I woke early the next morning. A dog was barking, a new voice. I closed my eyes, listened carefully, and figured out that it must be three doors up the block, in the piano mover's yard. That made sense. His dog had been killed chasing a cat across the street. Hit by a car. The piano mover had been mourning for months. But he'd told me, recently, that he was sure his dog would have wanted him to get another.

Certainties

At thirty Ralph wasn't really what you'd call a happy bachelor, though like many former husbands he'd gone after what he perceived to be greater freedom. His married friends at work envied him, and he played the game, just winking when they asked what he'd been doing the night before, why he was looking so worn out, but for nearly a year he rued his divorce. Chastised himself, catalogued the many wrongs he'd done his wife, tried finally to win her back, starting with flowers on her birthday. This though he'd in effect forced her to leave him, ever more curt and abrupt, verbally abusive, lacking the courage to come out and tell her he wanted a separation. His mourning, nonetheless, was as heartfelt as it was self-deceived.

Part of the problem was that he was alone too much. He had vast reaches of time to fill, almost daily had to plan what he'd do for an evening, for the coming weekend. Nothing just happened; everything became intentional. He feared if he stopped extending himself, making calls, getting out and around, he'd just spend another night, another weekend, by himself. Watching TV.

It took a while, but after that endless first year on his own he felt better. He'd enrolled in a cooking class to keep himself busy and now could prepare a range of interesting meals, could invite dates to join him for dinner at his place. He began to enjoy shopping, too, for the first time, deciding carefully what he'd have for dinner, where he could get the best produce, what wine would be appropriate. He put on weight and then began playing more tennis to keep himself in shape. He had to look good, care about himself. He also began to enjoy seeing different women, feeling privy to some larger mystery just by getting to know his lovers' idiosyncrasies. What gave pleasure; what the limits were. Who could have imagined? One woman served him steak and potatoes but liked him to dominate her sexually, pin her down and take her, so to speak, against her will. Another woman, with Michelangelo's Adam in the heavens above her bed, kept saying she wanted something permanent, but never suggested it should be him. Meeting these women and others, Ralph tried to suspend judgment: here at long last was the wide world; now he was part of it. He was learning something all the time.

He was bothered, though, that coupling seemed to have to precede friendship, if friendship in fact ensued. "I hope you can get it up," a woman he met at a bar said to him on the way to her place. And, often, waking beside a semistranger, Ralph felt he was sowing his seed at random. Not that he wanted children, or marriage again—God forbid!—but surely there could be some continuities. One night, going to see *Last Tango in Paris* with a woman he'd recently met, Ralph smiled as Brando thundered "no names, no names" at Maria Schneider, insisting that they know as little as possible about each other. Still amused by the hyperbole of the scene, Ralph suddenly realized that he couldn't think of his date's name. He struggled the rest of the movie to remember it. They spent the night together, and before falling off to sleep he planned to check her purse in the morning. She got up before him, however, and it wasn't until hours later at work that he finally remembered.

Though often flattered by his successes, sure that he understood women better all the time, several incidents persuaded Ralph that the single life wasn't for him. First, he slept several times with the wife of one of his tennis partners. He liked the man well enough—a decent person, a bit dull, but nobody's enemy. Nobody but his wife, that is. She took to dropping by Ralph's place, always to complain about her husband. Though it was clearly to Ralph's advantage to be sympathetic, he found it hard: she was pretty, but a shrew. When, one night, she said she wanted to stay over, Ralph could have been more enthusiastic. He simply fell asleep with her beside him, determined not to be forced to take on every woman who came his way, but by morning they were making love. Such as it was.

The next time they saw each other she asked him when he was leaving on his vacation to Hawaii. Though she and her husband were supposed to be going to the Sierras together, she said Ralph's plans sounded more appealing. Could she come along? Her husband wouldn't object, she assured him. Hearing this, a little high on white wine, Ralph sobered up fast. Was such weighing of small advantage all one could expect? Could he hope for more? Angrily, he told her he was going by himself. Which he knew he'd regret, since he'd be lonely the whole time.

Still chewing on all this several days later, he went to visit his friend Bruce. A confirmed bachelor for years, Bruce had the game down pat, presiding over sunbathing in his backyard and a small sauna he'd built in the basement. Indeed, Ralph considered Bruce a genius at getting women to undress. Part of his skill was in making nudity seem cosmopolitan, as if only a crude soul could find anything offensive in it or suspect some ulterior motive. What, indeed, could be more natural?

That particular afternoon Ralph was hoping to meet Bruce's new woman, since, untypically, Bruce was saying seriously that he was in love. As Ralph came down the driveway to the back yard, he caught sight of two naked bodies. Approaching closer, he could see Bruce hurriedly covering his lady friend with a robe. Protective, proprietary. The afternoon passed; Ralph never did see her naked. It gave him pause.

Finally, he came home from work one evening to find yet another note from a woman he'd met only once, at a party. Since then she'd been writing him almost daily or coming by to leave flowers, messages, love poems, small gifts. Loneliness had driven her crazy. Knowing almost nothing about him, she was certain he was the man she wanted. "Love is what's important, Ralph," this note began, "and I want you to know that I love you. As a human being you make sense to me intellectually, intuitively, and sexually. Why should we hold back? Time is short. Call me tonight." He didn't call. Her desperation, parodying his, only made him sad.

He was particularly susceptible to depression because he'd met a woman he was very attracted to. They'd gone out a few times and had wonderful lovemaking. She was a filmmaker, and he was fascinated by her interests and ambitions. But when he called her up to go out again, she said that she couldn't see him anymore.

"I like you," she told him, "and I had a great time in bed with you, but I'm emotionally overextended. I'm seeing someone already, and a man I used to live with is coming into town again. I just can't handle it all." Ralph wanted to protest, to tell her how much he liked her, but what she'd said sounded fair. And final.

Months later, thinking back to all this, Ralph sighed with relief: he'd fallen in love. Though Anna was a little young, still finishing college, he was sure she was all he wanted. The only problem was to win her. But even that went more easily than he could have hoped. They got drunk on Scotch and laughed all night the first time they went out, both swearing in the morning that they never touched hard liquor. Which was pretty much true until they got into it together. Ralph, in any case, kept asking her out, and Anna kept accepting. One of her former lovers frequently called, and occasionally she had long phone conversations with him when Ralph spent the evening at her place, but she said that she wasn't seeing him anymore, and apparently she wasn't.

Finally, a month after they met, Ralph and Anna were comfortable enough together to venture out of Berkeley. He'd told her about his old friend Gail, and, nearly three hundred miles of highway behind them, they pulled in the long dirt driveway. Easing down, they checked out Gail's beehives, goats, chickens, and ducks while she regaled them with tales of her belly-dance students and her performances in local bars.

"I'll bet you're a Sagittarius," Gail suddenly said to Anna.

"How did you know?" Anna asked, startled. "Did Ralph tell you?"

"He doesn't believe in the stars," Gail replied, "but all the women he's really loved have been Sagittarius."

This talk made Ralph uneasy. He felt too predictable, to begin with, nor did he like it said that he'd loved other women. Had Anna been put off, he wondered. Apparently not. As they moved into the house to inspect Gail's collection of thrift-shop Orientalia, their eyes met. Abruptly excusing themselves, hurriedly closing the door of the spare bedroom, they made sweet and noisy love for what seemed like hours. When they finally emerged, heading for the tub with a sheet around them to cover what was left of their modesty, Gail laughed. "I guess you two are sexually compatible," she said. "You're one lucky man, Ralph. You don't deserve her. But don't you just love his legs, Anna?"

"Did you spend time with Gail?" Anna asked when they were in the tub.

"We're old friends," Ralph said, begging the question.

"Were you lovers too?"

"A couple of times," Ralph answered reluctantly, afraid of what might follow.

"You have good taste. Gail's very beautiful. I'm glad we came up here."

"Good," Ralph said, enormously relieved. Maybe he never would understand women, he thought.

The next night, Gail out dancing, Ralph and Anna drove down to the beach north of Arcata. Walking a mile or so in the heavy fog, they pushed on, though both were tired, until Anna located a spot she deemed appropriate. Rejecting Ralph's suggestion of a hollow in some marsh grass on the edge of the dunes, carefully considering a driftwood fort (only to dismiss it when she noticed some beer cans nearby), she finally chose an enormous redwood stump that had washed down Mad River into Humboldt Bay. Cold wind whistling through their legs, bark damp beneath her, sand blowing on his back and behind, their bellies joined. They felt no pain.

Years later, well after they were safely married, when they had long since created between them a sorrow for nearly every joy, Ralph was nevertheless not nostalgic for the early days of their relationship: the state of falling in love had been nerve-racking. Just before that trip to Kneeland, for instance, they had a date to meet at his apartment at midnight. As usual, Anna planned to study at the library until closing time. At one, however, she had still not arrived. Ralph had told her several times that it was pointlessly dangerous to bike around Berkeley late at night, but she'd only laughed. "I can take care of myself," she'd told him.

Indeed, Ralph believed her, feared, in fact, that she was young enough and independent enough not to need him. Not as he needed her, in any case. Though as time passed he was increasingly anxious, phoning her apartment several times, he was not at all certain that his concern for her safety was warranted. To this point they were, obviously, lovers. But only that. Perhaps Anna had decided to be alone. Or to see someone else. The passion they shared seemed to give him no claim on her reliability, not to mention fidelity. It did seem totally out of character for her to be late, or for her not to call; they'd been together nearly every night since they'd met; but still he felt he had no real claim on her.

After calling her apartment every few minutes from one to one-thirty, Ralph decided to go over and take a look. In case her phone was out of order, he told himself, or because she might have stopped there and fallen asleep. Though aware that he might learn more than he wanted to, he went downstairs and got into his car. Following the route across town she usually biked, hoping to spot her, he saw only some stray dogs, several cats, and two street people with backpacks moving silently up to the hills to camp for the night.

When he reached her place no lights were on; his knocking drew no response. Jumping back in his car, he dismissed the thought that she'd been inside, listening. Running stop signs all the way back to his apartment, he took the stairs two at a time, hurried in the front door toward the phone—wondering if he was insane to be calling the police, or insane not to have called them sooner—and nearly jumped out of his skin when Anna leapt out from behind the bookcase as he rushed past.

Ralph could have throttled her. Not for scaring him, though she continued to laugh uncontrollably for several minutes at how startled he'd been, how successfully she'd surprised him. No, even after she explained that she was sure she'd told him the library was open late in exam period, he had to fight to control his rage. He kept seeing himself driving across town to her apartment: racking his brain to see if he'd said or done something to offend her; unsure of what he'd find, utterly unable to decide whether he should be sick with worry or wild at being treated so shabbily.

The night passed—ended with them curled in each other's arms—but he was left thinking that what they shared might be no more than ephemeral. Another affair. Desperate for substance, he pushed hard the next months to normalize their relationship, to be able to take it and her if not for granted, then as a given. Yet it was more than a year before he stopped believing that he had to be on his best behavior, that if he were "himself" Anna would have good reason to leave.

Ralph's quest for certainty, as it happened, took him through a number of emotional mine fields. Toward the end of their trip to Kneeland, very happy, for the first time he told her he loved her.

"Don't say that," she responded sharply.

"Why not?" he answered, hurt.

"I hate it. People use the word 'love' so carelessly. Everybody does."

"But I mean it."

"Maybe you do, but you don't have to tell me. When you say it, then I'm forced to say the same thing. And I don't like to."

"You don't love me?" he said too quickly, knowing as he heard himself that he'd willfully misread her, was being coercive.

"Did I tell you that? Can't you understand what I'm saying?"

"For Christ's sake," he muttered, unwilling not to have the last word, but feeling more precarious than ever.

On another occasion, snuggled dreamily next to her, Ralph said he hoped they'd be together forever. She laughed.

"Is that what you told your ex-wife?"

"What's she got to do with us?"

"It seems obvious."

"Not to me. That wasn't the same thing. Not at all."

"No?"

"I'm telling you no. I was much younger then. She's not you. She and I together weren't the same as we are together. I don't even want to think about it."

"*That* I can believe," Anna said.

Or, when from time to time Anna spoke of her travels in Greece and North Africa, Ralph always fell silent, wearing a hangdog expression that might have silenced someone less strong. When, finally, she called him on it, he tried humor but was obviously serious.

"Who wants to hear about your infidelities?" he said.

"Infidelities? You mean when I was with Rick?"

"I don't particularly want to hear his name, thank you."

"How was that unfaithful? Come on, explain yourself. How was I unfaithful when I was with Rick?"

"You weren't with me, were you."

"Of course not. We hadn't met."

"I know that."

"Then what? Should I have been waiting for you? Is that what you mean?"

"You could have thought about it, at least."

And then late one night, after they'd made love and were still drunk enough to be lapping Johnny Walker Black out of each other's navels, Anna asked him if he didn't mind "being imprisoned in monogamy." Ralph again felt an enormous gulf between them. Of course she was young, he thought. She'd want to try out a lot of different things. He barely slept that night.

Months passing, however, he learned to let her actions speak instead of the words he wanted to hear. Not so very hard, since most of the time they were happy together. Proud, he knew he was overcoming a failing in himself and was particularly satisfied with what he gleaned from rereading Saint-Exupery's *Le Petit Prince:* "S'il te plaît . . . apprivoise-moi," the fox tells the prince. "That's what it is," Ralph thought, earmarking the page. "She's just telling me how to tame her. Fair enough. Why didn't I understand?"

Despite his self-congratulation, it was perhaps simply the passage of time that made him feel more at ease. Slowly, shared history superseded the unknown; what they had between them now was grounded in specifics. And a past, particularly one full of pleasure, suggested to him that a not dissimilar future could be inferred. An innocent bystander might have poked holes in Ralph's logic, of course. Didn't he remember his first marriage? But his memory was selective. He felt good.

Since they were both now working, her studies completed, routine also gave him the pleasant sensation of predictability. Life had boundaries; even passion had to fit its forms. If this meant that their lovemaking slowly lost the abandon of their early days together, Ralph felt it was not too high a price to pay. Nothing was perfect, after all.

There was nonetheless one recurrent phenomenon which, though predictable, never failed to undermine his need for certainty. Whenever he and Anna were separated for any substantial length of time, more than a week, say, at the moment they were reunited it was—it seemed to him—almost as if they were strangers. They always recognized each other, never for a moment stopped being man and wife, but always he felt Anna merely going through the motions of greeting him, holding her body back, her embrace only formal. Each time, miles successfully spanned, after phone calls every day, a vast distance remained to be closed.

It was just once, after their first separation when he visited his family by himself, that Ralph carried Anna up to bed as soon as they reached home, insisting by his actions that intimacy was of course in order. From that time on, however, whenever they were reunited hours would pass before they made love, the small familiarities of the prosaic finally reinforcing a sense of shared lives. But even then, like animals checking scents before mating, they would move warily toward each other.

Always this made Ralph feel that what bound them was, after all, quite fragile. And, further, that it had been some deception on his part, or some kind of psychological violence, that had domesticated Anna. He had, obviously, pursued her relentlessly, leaving her no time or space to be with anyone else. He'd contrived every kind of pleasure for them he could: long walks on the pier on the Bay; hikes in the hills; visits to a friend's place at Stinson Beach; good meals at Japanese restaurants with lots of sake; films. And their lovemaking. Of course their pleasure in each other had astonished them both. But often, when they could easily have slept, he'd come in her again, once more bringing her to climax, as if, were her pleasure great enough, she would lose all reason. And want to stay with him.

Or, Ralph often thought, coercion aside, if she had in fact committed herself with what could be called her own free will, then she just hadn't been able to foresee the consequences. Perhaps because he withheld the truth. When they first met, for one thing, Anna didn't realize he was napping after work each day to be able to sustain their all-night lovemaking. In a confessional mood some months later, Ralph told her, and he was amazed that she didn't feel defrauded. Similarly, after he proposed he told her that she could make a better match. She simply stared at him, stared until he felt compelled to defend himself. "I'm older than you are, Anna. I know about these things."

They had nonetheless married, and five years together brought them a not abnormal mix of pleasures and pains, though probably less strife than many couples experience. She compulsively complained about his driving, to the point that Ralph often threatened to run them into a pole. But late at night she'd search his skin for blemishes, like a chimp delousing its mate. He nagged her almost daily about not closing doors behind her, or not dressing up enough, but frequently said how happy she made him, and often soaped her back when she took a bath.

In that fifth year, however, Ralph began to complain that they weren't making love often enough, though he'd long since found such direct challenges counterproductive: Anna simply got her hackles up. Still, he couldn't stop himself, perhaps because one night she'd asked him if he wasn't bored with her sexually after so long together. He had thought many times that he'd take lovers if he weren't afraid of losing her; he understood that she might just be searching for a compliment or some affection; but her words unsettled him. Her question suggested the possibility of enormous changes, and who knew what would happen? Thinking it over later, he concluded she was really saying he didn't satisfy her anymore.

On this slim evidence he built his case; that same night he began to argue it. Telling her again and again that all *he* needed was real responsiveness from her, though of course he couldn't speak for what she was after. As he could have predicted, Anna only grew more remote, while he felt like a fool for trying to bludgeon her with accusations into, as he'd put it, "being more loving." Yet he persisted. He couldn't stop himself. He slept alone that night on the living room couch.

The three following nights he also slept alone, and poorly, angry at her, angry at himself. He was tired of women, he told himself over and again. Tired of being with them, tired of being afraid of being without them. After five years with Anna, after his time as a bachelor, after his first marriage, he was sick of making things work, worrying they wouldn't work. Exhausted with all the possibilities, all the ambiguities. His needs, his responses. He wanted an end to it; didn't want to be reasonable anymore; didn't want to understand; didn't want someone understanding him. For once in his life, he kept telling himself, he just wanted things his way. Period.

Still on the living room couch that fifth night, he kept thinking how incredible it would be to once and for all end Anna's capacity for withdrawal. For disagreement, for change. He lost more sleep fantasizing victories over her. Taking a lover, someone with the kind of olive complexion she always envied. Watching Anna beg him to come home. Refusing to go to bed with her when, crying, she tried to make it up to him. Spurning her apologies again and again.

As their war of attrition went a sixth, seventh, and then an eighth day, however, Anna gave every sign of being able to outlast him. "She doesn't need me," he thought morosely. "She doesn't even need to fuck. She could go on this way for years. For centuries."

"You have to woo me and win me," Anna said, laughing, on the ninth night. Right in the middle of his complaints, as though he was just being foolish. Though now nearly exhausted, he worked himself into another rage. He'd get her to acknowledge she was wrong, somehow he would. He'd show her. But later that night, confronting the living room couch yet another time, he made a series of bleak admissions to himself. One: he'd be better off alone, but wouldn't be able to stand it. Two: without him she'd flourish, and his best friends would be the first to come around. And three—most bitter of all: he just was never really going to get his way.

Full of self-pity, his mind spinning with resentment, he paced around the house until he finally settled at the kitchen table. Still looking out the breakfast-nook window into the blackness at three-thirty, utterly spent, he heard a door open upstairs. Several moments later Anna came into the kitchen.

"What are you doing up so late?" she asked, a thin, but not tight, smile on her lips.

"What do you think?" He studied her smile, trying to figure out what it was for. She didn't dare believe she'd won, did she?

"I'm sure I don't know." Still smiling.

Now Ralph was up against it. Was he going to keep fighting for some acknowledgment that he'd been right all along? Or, after nine nights, was he going to bite the bullet? Worse than that—woo her and win her. Otherwise, if things kept on going, one of them, probably him, was going to have to pack up and take off. Oops. There was the void again. Scary. Very scary.

He stared at Anna. Still that same smile. Inviting, he had to admit. She looked good, very good indeed. No wonder everyone told him he was lucky to have her. He certainly wanted to hold her, to open her robe and kiss her breasts, to have her holding him. Christ, he wanted her.

"It's late," Ralph said, noncommittally. Pleased at how long he'd let the silence run, how long Anna had been standing there. Smile or not. Congratulating himself for not having given away any more. Maybe he could still salvage something.

"It certainly is," she said.

There was another long silence. He thought of several strategies, options, possibilities. What to say, with what inflection, at what speed. With what tone of voice. The choices were tough.

"I've been acting a little crazy, I guess, lately," he finally said, throwing in the "lately" at the last possible moment to add some ambiguity. And then, not satisfied, continuing on. "Not sleeping enough, probably, that must be part of it." There, he'd said it. A mixed bag. She'd have to make of it what she could. She'd have to take it or leave it. And if that smile turned smug he'd stay up all night just to show her he wasn't finished. Not by a long shot.

Her response, which he listened to very carefully, was—and he analyzed every nuance—"Let's go to bed." He gave her a long searching look, weighed her words another time. She smiled again. He got up. No irretrievable commitment yet. Or was there? Quite suddenly, it seemed to him, though it could have happened at normal speed, she turned, crossed the kitchen, and headed for the doorway.

His move now, but with very limited options. Very limited indeed, he thought. Alone, on his feet, he shook his head. Grinned foolishly. Shrugged his shoulders. Said, out loud, "Fuck it." There really was no point: one way or the other, he'd just have to follow her up the stairs.

Waiting Till Thirty

Mid-winter, bitter cold and absolutely clear, snow drifted high on the frozen ground. Occasional cars ghosting by, or one trying to rock free, tires whining for traction.

"We met almost six years ago," he's saying, sipping his drink as we sit by the fire. "Just after you went west. It's funny. People considered us the ideal couple, and in a way I thought we were. I'd watched so many of my friends' weddings just after college, and then I'd seen all the bickering and the divorces. I thought, turning thirty, that I was ready, that it would be different. I'd reached some sense of myself and what I wanted, and I knew what my career would look like. In any event, we met, married, and had the two kids. We both wanted them. Life was hectic but good. I was working hard at teaching and on the book. She was caring for the kids and finishing her master's.

"Then about a year and a half ago we started having trouble. 'When we go to parties,' she told me, 'I find myself telling your jokes, talking about your work, thinking what you think.' I tried to argue with her, but it wasn't easy. One might have said that this is what it is to know someone well. I could have told her that I also spoke about her a lot. But what she was saying was true, became more important than the other truths between us. She just needed to be on her own. I'd never considered that possibility. I knew that I had waited a long time to get married. She won't even be twenty-eight until next spring.

"Anyway, it went on for a while without being resolved, and then she saw a small house across town for sale. Now we share the kids, and things are peaceful between us. Nor can I say I'm totally cast adrift. We still value each other, and what with my teaching, the writing, and the kids, life is okay. And around here there are all kinds of women looking for eligible men."

We sit silent for a moment. I never imagined that he was in danger of being "totally cast adrift," but his phrase gives me pause. I look around once again. The house, which she had begun to remodel, remains unfinished, walls stripped but not repainted, bricks waiting to be made into a hearth. And, kids at her place tonight, the house is just too big, more than he needs.

It grows dark; the wind picks up. There's a draft coming through the old floorboards. "I have to put down some linoleum," he says apologetically. Despite the fire, we both feel the chill.

The Price of Song

Startling, the enormous valley far below, an almost-mirage sighted from the high country of the Sierras, a vast bowl perhaps twenty by ten miles. At its eastern verge a crossroads ranching community, population two hundred, elevation five thousand feet. Two cafés, a general store, post office, and grade school. Perhaps thirty homes, many owned by offspring of the Italian-Swiss who came to find gold but stayed on to log and work cattle. Immigrants whose arrival terminated the annual summer migration of Indian bands to the valley, their traditional trek up from winter camps in the foothills.

Summer in the valley. A short growing season, too brief for most fruits and vegetables, killing frosts early and late. Powerful sun blasting stillness into each endless day, until, long overdue, a rising west wind rustles the leaves of cottonwoods towering over homes in town and farmhouses remote on the plain. Nights cold; floorboards chilling bare soles in the morning. Ground fog engulfing all but the very peaks of the barns' pitched roofs.

Summer. Early and late the sound, often from miles across the bowl, of logging-truck gears being double-clutched; or the rattles of an old pickup just down the way. Cattle fattening for market, wood being corded, all scheduled against the coming winter. Lightning storms, hard rain, hail. Cumulus clouds paralleling the valley floor, so close and seeming substantial that one could climb just a few rungs of Jacob's ladder to walk that higher plateau. Keeping an eye out, of course, for patches of cirrus.

Summer. Bats after sunset sweeping back and forth near the houses as if begging to be admitted. And a hummingbird, trapped inside, beating all night against the pane.

This very small community, still often unreachable for days during the winter, even in fair weather nearly an hour from the county seat. Off the tourist track: no lakes, no skiing, no Victorian storefronts. A hard place when it was settled. *Emma. Died June 1, 1896. Age 22 years and 4 months. Also our twin sons Edward and Erwin. Age 3 weeks.* And still a hard place, the low taxes and quiet notwithstanding, despite the good hunting and creek fishing. Winters just too damn severe. No work anywhere, particularly with the log mills shutting down. Too many old people. Always a backwater, but now without a promise even of continuing what was. A future only in rumors—scientologists planning to buy the old Vinelli place down the road; golf course developers evisioning the valley as one enormous fairway.

It must have been thirty-five summers ago, not long after World War II, that young Albert House and his bride Mildred first passed through town with a logging gang, mostly his brothers and cousins. The men cut, she cooked and cleaned. They lived in tents in the mountains and stayed until snow threatened. Then, following the rhythms of Albert's people, headed down to the foothills.

The next summer Mildred found a place to rent on the outskirts of town. Albert refused to let her come up to the mountains again: the crew was too rowdy this year, he said; he'd be afraid for her. Each Sunday he came in from camp to leave his dirty clothes and pick up the food she'd prepared. Loaves and loaves of bread. Cakes, doughnuts, dried fish, dried fruit. Sometimes he'd bring down a deer he'd taken out of season, leaving it with her to dress and jerk.

Mildred was in that house nearly four months and just about went insane. Each day she walked to the store and back, maybe two miles in all, always buying something—butter, thread, a candle, fishhooks—but often doing so only to justify her trip. She needed human contact; the isolation was driving her mad. Each day she'd walk slowly, very slowly, along the unpaved shoulder of the road, looking for anything that might be a distraction. A rancher baling hay, neck burning, massive belt buckle disappearing under paunch. A coyote crossing the field, bold as you please. A turkey vulture wheeling, soaring higher, red skullcap leading the spirals.

Each of these empty days, four months' worth, Mildred passed the silent and staring locals sitting on their front porches under the cottonwoods and willows. None of them ever said a word to her: no one wanted to speak to the white woman who was married—she said!—to that Indian fella.

As they were packing up that autumn, Albert saw a notice on the telephone pole outside the general store, an announcement of a job opening at the grade school in town. Wanting year-round employment, realizing that if he logged long enough he'd lose a leg or his life, Albert went in to talk to the school-district man. And, to his surprise, got the job, scored higher on the test than the other applicants. "Custodian, Step One": salary, such as it was, every two weeks, fifty-two weeks a year; pension; health and insurance benefits. As Albert likes to say, still grinning after countless repetitions of the line over the years, he's been at school ever since.

Summers are the slow time, polishing floors, repainting walls. When school's in session, kids in perpetual motion, he settles for keeping the classrooms, corridors, and bathrooms clean, or moving furniture around. Setting up folding chairs in the auditorium/gymnasium for assemblies, then clearing it completely and lowering the backboards for basketball games. He also drives the school bus, circumnavigating the valley twice each weekday. Starting out at five-thirty, after milking, returning twelve hours later. Time for milking again.

Their own children are long gone now, and, with Albert at school so much, Mildred tends to wake late. In no hurry to face the day, chain-smoking as soon as she's up, turning on the TV, she drinks cup after cup of black coffee. She eats in the morning if at all, for despite the array of platters she sets on the table for Albert or for guests, no one ever sees her take a bite. If with his black hair and smooth weathered skin Albert seems more fifty than nearly sixty, Mildred—gaunt, face incredibly wrinkled—carries the weight of all her years.

Perhaps life with Albert wore her out. Not that he's a bad man, quite the contrary; nor is he a hard husband. He's always been willing to go out and work, has "always done what had to be done," as Mildred puts it. But early on he knew he'd have to fight. Stood next to his brothers and cousins as a child, taking on attackers; traded punches and kicks after tackles when he played football in high school; more than once stepped outside the bar to settle things when he was in the service. Fought to win Mildred. It may be that, so much behind him so soon, he accepted what people can be like. Acquired early on a certain bemused tolerance for their stupidities and cruelties. Or perhaps just exerted tremendous self-control, imposing will on a natural taciturnity. Watching and waiting. Never letting on, possibly even to himself, exactly what he felt.

But not Mildred. Raised by her grandparents, at an early age she was taking cattle to the back country on her own, spending days out there. She could ride, brand, doctor animals, repair fences, take care of just about anything. Though she had to tell her grandfather to go to hell when he objected to Albert, she was used to being able to improve something, make a change, work it out. Prejudice, however, bamboozled her.

Even Albert's name gave her trouble. *House.* What could be more ordinary, more prosaic? Less Indian. Albert said he'd never thought about it, had no idea where the name came from. It was just there, a word. But when Mildred first came to the valley, every time her signature was required—to register to vote; at the doctor's; at the electric company; at the hospital the day she broke her hand—every time, she'd see the clerk's face change, as if she had somehow tried to deceive them. Hell, they knew better, she was the Indian's wife. As if Albert should be wearing loincloth and feathers and calling himself Sitting Bull. *House!* She came to hate the name, but what could you do?

Actually, short of changing it, she and Albert did quite a bit, all they could. Sometimes, looking back over the years, reappraising one of the countless small victories, Mildred marvels at what they achieved. They could have lived down in the foothills with his people or kept to themselves in the valley, but instead, never discussing it together, not once, they determined to win the respect of those who held them in contempt. And, on the basis of that respect, to be accepted.

For instance, once they settled in the valley Albert never again took a drink. Not just hard liquor, either, but, even after cutting firewood on a stinking hot day, sweat running down through the grime on his chest, horseflies biting, never even a sip of beer. He just wasn't going to be the drunken Indian, or give anyone room to suggest he was. In sympathy, though Albert never spoke of it, Mildred stopped using alcohol too. They'd both be beyond reproach.

The achingly slow process of acceptance: in unspoken accord, Albert and Mildred kept at it. At the local store they made it a point not to run up a bill. Each and every time, they paid cash, just to show they could take care of themselves. Not like some others, as Mildred often said. To supplement Albert's small salary, Mildred worked part-time as a waitress, also baking the café's pies. They always managed to set a little more money aside.

After Albert had been at the school three years, a storeowner in the market town on the far side of the valley suggested that they take advantage of the special price he was offering on new refrigerators. Mildred really wanted one, but Albert told the man they just didn't have enough saved up. "You got a job, don't you?" the man asked. "Over at the primary school?" Albert nodded. "Well, then," the man said, "as I see it, you're a whole lot better off than most around here. I don't mind carrying the loan. Not one bit."

Mildred often tells this story, always as if it was some special act of generosity to allow them to pay eighteen percent on the note. "I still put flowers on his grave," she says, fiercely. "I'll be doing it until the day I die, too, if I have my way."

Later, when this same man became the Ford dealer, he told them they deserved a better vehicle. Soon Albert was driving over on the first of each month—proud of his new pickup—with money for both payments in his wallet.

Slowly, slowly, they became part of the community. Got a bank loan for a home. Worked to keep lawns neat, trim painted, wood corded cleanly. Lots of wood, for that matter, sometimes fifteen cords out back. "To show we weren't afraid of work, that we were the kind that planned ahead," Mildred says. And, on the chance that someone would come by to visit or, on the pretext of a visit, to snoop, Mildred kept the house spotless, going over it again and again until every surface sparkled, until Albert complained that there wasn't a place dirty enough for him to step or sit down on.

Through these years, Mildred always thanked God that the nearest reservation was seventy miles away. It would be easier, she was sure, for people to relate to Albert as an individual. And she was glad he worked at the school, drove the kids. People got to see him around, had to concede he did a good job, clearly enjoyed the children. But still it wasn't easy. Every year the principal had the teachers for dinner. There were just two teachers, Albert the only other adult in the school. Though as years passed teachers came and went, though Albert was always there, the principal never invited him to come. Mildred never stopped believing that the new year would be different; Albert never spoke about it.

Far from passively hoping for change, however, Mildred did everything in the community she possibly could. Baked for the various Grange sales, bazaars, and picnics. Visited the sick and elderly; gave blood; brought blankets, clothing, and food to the victims of flood and fire. It took time, but the local women, seeing her efforts, began to invite her to participate. Mildred knew they spoke against her behind her back, even whispered that she wasn't really married to Albert, but she realized they did that kind of thing to each other. At least they were calling her.

The children were another blessing. Mildred never had any, and if over time she made peace with the fact, she perceived that to be childless set her apart from the other women in town, made it harder to share their lives or conversations. But then Albert's brother and sister-in-law died in a car crash, and they decided to take in the three boys. Mildred loved them as her own, but also never minded at all that they made her seem more normal, even if everyone in the valley knew just how they'd come to her. And, fortunately, they were obedient kids, better-than-average students, fine athletes. One even became vice-president of his class at high school. Mildred was certain that her strict discipline was at least part of the reason the boys did so well. Not like so many of the other kids.

Albert, meanwhile, had himself found some acceptance, invited after about eight years of working at the school to join the local sportsmen's club. Though he had stopped hunting by this time, Albert enjoyed the monthly meetings, the pounding of the gavel, the parliamentary protocol, seeing his name in the mimeographed newsletter they printed up each month with the minutes of the meeting. "Albert House suggested the deer quota should be increased this year on account of the heavy rains last fall." Or, "Albert House says the old logging road to Mill Lake should be graded or shut down otherwise, since even four-wheel drive can't get you through those mud slides."

In time, in fact, Albert was elected treasurer of the club. His picture appeared in the valley weekly, a shot of him dressed, as always, in a green Sears work shirt (top of a white T-shirt visible at the collar) and green work pants, tips of his cowboy boots protruding from under the cuffs. His mouth slightly open, not to talk but, as usual, to listen. Oh, Albert says things to people, and not just at club meetings. But it's remarkable how little a man has to speak to get by. The talkers always talk anyway, their salutations almost invariably the same, barely requiring a verbal response. A smile, particularly from a man understood to be both gentle and quiet, does it all.

"Hey, Albert, how's it going?"

"Kids ganging up on you, Albert, that why you're looking so whupped?"

"Hell, Albert, if I was you I'd risk a speeding ticket just once in that damn school bus. Crank her up and see what she'll do, for God's sake."

"What's new, Albert? How's Mildred?"

Now long since accepted, Albert seems essentially unchanged. Still laconic, still smiling, though his reserve as always leaves one to speculate on what he really feels. But particularly when one sees him with the school kids or at work around the house, he seems a man satisfied with what he does, where he finds himself; a man without terrible scars. And Mildred? "Oh, those hippies," she says, lighting another cigarette. "I heard they're back at the hot springs, running around naked, doing God knows what. Right out in plain view. Some people have no shame. I hope the sheriff gets down there quick and moves them on. Or else. They're offending a lot of decent people, people who live here."

At some level, Mildred surely remembers swimming naked with Albert up in the small freezing lakes where they logged, laughing as he chased her through the reeds and mud and pulled her down. Neither of them worrying, at those moments, about mosquitoes or leeches. Mildred also knows that no one has gone near the springs for years except to make love in the back seat of a car, that if anyone can see the hippies they'd have to have driven over to take a look. But she's said this kind of thing far too many times. Her words have a life of their own, and live it.

So Mildred's down on hippies. Votes Republican and tells you why. (Too much government interference. Too many laws. Russians getting too powerful. Bureaucrats spending money on the kind of people who won't help themselves.) She was truly sad to see Reagan leave office, would vote for him again. Any time, any place.

More, she has a sharp word for the loose men and women in town, particularly the divorcées. Did they think it would be all roses? Is that what they figured? They just didn't try hard enough to make the marriage work, did they? And what about all the drinking going on? And the kids? Running wild, not like they used to. Need more discipline, that's what they need. A little discipline never hurt anybody, did it?

And the new Indian movement? Well, particularly in recent years Mildred has made sure everyone remembers that Albert is an Indian, has even claimed a little Indian blood for herself. Not long ago she put several Washoe baskets on the mantle, some Pueblo concho belts and Plains Indian beadwork up there too. A Navajo rug on the floor. And when a Western is on TV she watches it critically, quick to tell guests that of course that wasn't the way it was at all. "But these militants," she says, "occupying that island and things like that. Shooting at the police. That's not right. They should watch out. They'll get the taxpayer mad, and then where will they be? I ask you. Who's going to bail them out then?" Albert, who has forgotten all but a very few words of his people's tongue, sits silent.

By staying on so long in the valley even as the town has been dying, Albert and Mildred have outlived many of their adversaries to assume a position of importance in the tiny community, in part because there simply is no one else. The children of most of the Italian-Swiss families are long gone, and though Albert and Mildred are relative newcomers, they are at least old enough to understand the world of the remaining ranchers, to have been shaped by it. Just down the road from their place, Ed Martini still lives on his enormous ranch. But he's crippled, and his wife is perennially ailing. They don't like nurses around, so the Houses—as neighbors, as people who have known them a long time—help out. Fetch the firewood, shovel the snow, bring in the mail. If for years

Martini and his wife made no overtures, treated Albert and Mildred as though they didn't exist, now things are different. It almost seems that Albert and Mildred were always the Martinis' friends.

For seventeen years Albert has milked his cow Juniper twice a day, and recently, since he's at the Martinis' so much, he keeps her in their barn. Someone else could of course do the milking, but Albert thinks he should. Juniper knows him. Albert could also let her dry up: neither he nor Mildred drinks milk—digestion troubles—and he usually can't even give it away. But, needed at Juniper's side morning and evening, the farthest he's gone in seventeen years is day-hunting or over to the county fair.

Each time, he enters the barn through the windowless anteroom where milk used to be stored. Like many ranch structures in the valley, it's in disrepair, light filtering through gaps in the roof. Coming into the central portion of the barn, a vast room perhaps sixty feet high, Albert walks along the string of stalls. Forking some hay into the manger, Albert opens a side door for Juniper, who's been waiting, lowing, outside. Though she must be twenty, she's fat and glossy, her hide still shines. By this time all the cats and kittens, some four families, have gathered up from their hiding places under the floorboards. Juniper goes right into her stall and starts eating. The cats wait. Squatting beside Juniper on the milking stool, Albert slides in the pail, and, a dug between each thumb and forefinger, quickly milks her dry with firm rhythmic pulls.

Pail foaming, he pours perhaps a gallon of milk into various bowls, which he places in different spots in the hope that all the cats will get some. Then, though as always Juniper would prefer to stay and eat, Albert shoos her out the door. Getting back into his pickup, Albert drives the three hundred yards up to his place. He could walk, of course, but few men in town walk when they can drive. And Albert is proud of his new truck, its winch and oversize cab. Working at school so much, he just doesn't get to use it enough.

Home again, he puts another log in the stove and turns on the TV. The Olympics are on, a young Russian girl walking the balance beam, an American boy holding an iron cross on the rings. During the ads Albert turns away from the screen, not wanting, he says, to fill his head with garbage. "I like to let my mind wander," he explains. But how far? Mildred lights yet another cigarette, talks on the phone to her best friend about the upcoming benefit for the volunteer fire department, their conversation moving quickly to the latest local scandals. Tuning her out too, looking at the waxed floors, no dust visible, does Albert think of the cabin he was raised in, accessible only by foot, with its packed dirt floors and handmade shingles? Where he and his brother were horses, tin cans for hooves, switches for tails?

It's never easy to tell what Albert is thinking: he's passed most of a life without saying. And besides, the commercial is over. If, lips parted, Albert wasn't just listening to the announcer's voice, if, looking past the plaque he received for twenty-five years of service at the school, he was about to speak, now he keeps his thoughts to himself. As he always has.

All Concerned

Both twenty-five, Paul and Charlotte had been lovers for several years and shared a big house with Charlotte's best friend Karen and her husband. When Paul and Karen found themselves falling in love, they tried to fight it but then declared their feelings and moved into an apartment. Though Charlotte nearly went crazy, she finally recovered. Karen's husband left town.

The Christmas of the fourth year of their relationship, Paul and Karen went on vacation with their friends Mel and Betty. Paul and Betty, as it happened, were already lovers, though both felt unclean about their duplicity. Several months later Betty left Mel, and, soon after, Paul left Karen. Initially determined to live alone, Betty later decided to move in with Paul. Karen never realized that Paul and Betty had been lovers before the separations but, eager to be on her own, might not have much cared. Mel, however, threatened Betty and slashed a tire on Paul's car before giving up. A year later he remarried.

Karen remained close to Paul and Betty. After dating a number of men and enjoying her new freedom, she took up with Lee. They frequently saw Rob, who began to date Charlotte, Paul's former lover. Karen and Charlotte again became good friends. Now considering themselves feminists, they agreed that men shouldn't be allowed to disrupt the solidarity of sisterhood, and toyed with having an affair. But then Lee and Charlotte fell in love and decided to live together.

Karen was consoled by Betty and Paul, who, after two years, were having their own troubles. The relationship under stress, remembering how they'd found each other, they became wary of other couples, friends in particular. When Karen regained some confidence and expressed interest in Rob, both Betty and Paul were supportive. Taking the measure of the misery experienced by the various jilted mates in their circle, each concluded that such a solution, so obvious, would more than once have been best for all concerned.

Let Nature Take Its Course

In high school Jack got by on sheer luck, God only knows how. The girl he was going steady with looked, his closest friend told him knowingly, as if you could blink and she'd conceive. Not until they made love the first time, after a year's passionate everything-but, did Jack, shuddering involuntarily as he pulled up his pants, recall his friend's words. She was eager to get married, too, an aspiration which perhaps assuaged her fear of pregnancy.

Amazingly—and happily, as far as Jack was concerned—nothing happened. Though no longer "pure," as she put it, she still wore the gold circle pin Jack had given her. But when spring came, instead of announcing their engagement they quarreled. She accused him of wanting her only for sex, and, though he protested that she was wrong, they broke up just before the prom. Even then Jack sensed that he'd been spared.

His first semester of college, in 1960, he got off to a good start, doing well on his hour exams and meeting lots of girls at the dances held on campus each week. Around winter exam time, however, just when he should have been in the library cramming morning to night, he began to date a woman who worked as a research assistant for one of his professors. Nearly twenty-five, she seemed to Jack incredibly mature. Far from being a student, she'd dropped out long since, explaining to Jack that one could of course accomplish more outside academic routines. Indeed, she hardly had time to pursue her various interests. "I just can't allow myself to read periodicals," she told Jack, who, seldom having ventured past the sports page of the local daily, nodded knowingly.

Their first night together they went out to dinner. Normally voluble, Jack sat silent as she spoke about Mozart, Bach, Mann, civil rights, the Rosenberg case, Chagall. He recognized the names but couldn't, so to speak, place the faces. At her apartment later, as they listened to some John Fahey, she rolled what he thought was a cigarette, inhaled deeply, and offered it to him. "No, thank you, I don't smoke," he said, not realizing that she was passing a joint.

It was by this time nearly midnight, and Jack was agonizing about the studying he should have been doing. His friends would just now be packing up their notes, signing out reserve books to take to their rooms, planning to be back at the library when it opened at eight. He'd flunk out, he thought. Finally, heart beating from anxiety about unread pages, he said he thought he should go. Instead of getting his coat and walking him to the door, however, she embraced him, kissed him very gently, and guided his right hand between her legs.

If all this surprised Jack—he'd taken her out on a dare from his roommate, who'd bet she wouldn't accept, much less spend the night with him—he was startled when she suddenly pushed his hand away. Had he done something wrong?

"I have to put the diaphragm in," she said.

"What?" Jack said, associating the word with gym class and correct posture.

"My diaphragm. Unless you have some better idea."

"Oh, no," Jack answered, hoping he sounded nonchalant, watching her carefully as she took a small plastic case from her purse and went into the bathroom.

"All set," she said when she returned, now wearing a bathrobe. As they began to make love, Jack wondered what she'd done. It took some discreet inquiry, but by the end of exams he had a fair idea.

That summer Jack went to France and had the good fortune to meet an Austrian girl. Conversation, unfortunately, was limited: he spoke no German, she only halting English. What words they could exchange were in French, which they were both there to study.

Jack understood her intentions well enough that first night, however, to head down the four flights of stairs two at a time to find a pharmacy. Entering the store out of breath, he waited until the few customers left and then pretended to be browsing, hoping the proprietor's wife would go in the back room. Finally Jack walked up to the counter.

"Je vous en prie," he began. He liked the phrase anyway, and this time, he thought, he really had something to beg of someone. But even as the words left his mouth he realized that he lacked the crucial noun. *Condom?* Just didn't sound as if it would translate well. Certainly not *frenchy* or *French letter.* He'd heard that, returning the English compliment, the French called them *capots anglais,* but wasn't sure this was true.

What to say? The proprietor was still waiting. Cognates. Over and again Jack had been amazed at how well they worked. Administration? Nothing to it: *l'administration.* But in this case nothing came to mind, until, suddenly, he had a flash of inspiration: prophylactic. A ringing polysyllable, certainly deriving from Latin, probably surfacing in all Romance languages. A good risk. All he had to do was give it a little twist at the end for the sake of phonetics. "Je vous en prie," he began again, now with some confidence. "Est-ce que vous avez des prophylactiques?"

The proprietor just stared at him, clearly didn't understand. Jack looked around the store again in the faint hope that some would be on display, but of course not, not in this Catholic country. Not, in 1961, even in the States. His eyes met the proprietor's. An impasse. Several interminable—in French, *interminable*—moments went by. But then, conspiratorially, the man looked over his shoulder toward the back room, as if to make certain that his wife was out of hearing. Raising his eyebrows questioningly, making sure he had Jack's full attention, he extended the forefinger of his right hand and drove it savagely through a circle formed by the thumb and forefinger of his left.

Jack nodded vigorously. "Pré-serv-a-tif," the man enunciated, as if teaching a language class. Jack repeated it, grinning, pleased with success, the prospects of the evening, and the linguistic sense of it all.

Later that summer, though they had used the prophylactics

he purchased that night and quite a few more, the Austrian girl missed her period. Now the croissants and petits fours tasted less sweet; the professor's orations on the existentialists failed to impress; they stopped memorizing lists of new words. What were they going to do? Days passed; they waited. And then one morning as she stood by the bidet, she started laughing. "Jack, Jack, je ne suis pas avec ta babée," she shouted, unconcerned about the nosy concierge, utterly without interest in searching her mind for the correct idiom.

By the time Jack finished college he'd spent time with a number of women, considered himself a freethinker, frequently said he believed in free love. By this he meant sex without obligation, physical pleasure not burdened with what he liked to call "outmoded beliefs." These were high aspirations, to be sure, but often he found himself still hemmed in by the dead hand of the past. Once, for instance, he spent the night with a woman he met at a party. When they woke in the morning, painfully hung over, she accused him of having gotten her drunk to seduce her. This kind of accusation, however, like the issue of loss of reputation, disappeared as quickly as the risk of pregnancy when the Pill came into use. Just in time for the madness of the mid-sixties, if, as Jack often speculated, the Pill hadn't caused it all. So quick were the changes that soon Jack could hardly remember those "outmoded beliefs." Hadn't there been a time—no more than a moment ago—when he'd had to talk women into going to bed, when at least the charade of male as aggressor had been required? It was a new world, Jack thought; the game had changed.

Within a few years, however, other effects of the Pill had been catalogued. Nausea, bloating, vomiting, high blood pressure, headaches, blood clots. And IUD's, another technological wonder, could be expelled, or cause bleeding, cramps, pelvic infection.

It had been nice while it lasted, Jack thought; all he could have asked for and then some. But, on the other hand, so many private and public passions were playing themselves out. World turning, after such freedom he himself began to yearn for some limits, for something certain. Spending time with a woman he liked very much, he wanted to invest more in what they had between them, didn't want to share her affection or attention—not to mention her body—with anyone else. Became downright possessive, and liked it when she said she felt the same about him.

Whatever he'd once believed, he saw no anomalies when he asked her to marry him.

If for Jack promiscuity was now something of the past, he had still to confront the problem of contraception. His wife had gotten off the Pill soon after they started seeing each other ("too dangerous," she said) and stopped using the Dalkon Shield shortly before it was banned by the FDA. They were left, accordingly, to consider the alternatives short of celibacy. Neither liked diaphragms, and that was that. They tried spermicides for a while, but the foam, a mighty deterrent to oral-genital sex, burned her vagina. They read up on postcoital contraception, but this too seemed to have dangerous side effects. Jack could have solved the problem with a vasectomy, had friends who boasted of theirs, but he was, finally, reluctant to tamper with his manhood. Further, thinking that he might want children some day, he refused to trust a sperm bank. What if the refrigeration broke down?

Having determined that coitus interruptus was no more than a variation on Russian roulette, they were down to prophylactics and the rhythm method. They used the prophylactics, which neither of them much liked, whenever they thought she might be ovulating. This could have worked reasonably well, except that her periods were wildly irregular. Calculating safe days was difficult, conservative reckoning mandatory. In an attempt to be more precise, Jack's wife charted her daily body temperature over a number of cycles but concluded that early ovulation is always possible, that one knows only in retrospect when it has taken place. Not surprisingly, Jack became a frequent purchaser of Trojans, ruled a bathroom-cabinet domain of Sheiks and Rameses.

Thinking about the precautions necessary to avoid impregnating his wife, Jack occasionally asked himself the obvious question—why not children? For many years the answer had seemed absurdly simple. Children meant settling down, a loss of freedom. Jack had wanted to live his life a while, see what he thought of it, make choices, before continuing the cycle. If at all. Even in the sixties, when some considered making babies a wondrous affirmation of the life force, Jack held back, though there had been women who asked nothing more of him as potential father than his sperm.

When Jack met his wife he was thirty-one, she twenty-four. She told him several times before they married that she'd probably never want children. Having worked as a governess during college, she had no illusions about how much time and care children required, how the world could diminish to their scale. "If we have money for a nanny," she said, "I might do it. Or if you want to stay home and raise a child. But otherwise, I don't think so." Though what she said had both conviction and reason, Jack tended to discount her words. Whether it was culture or biology that had such force, he'd met too many women who, turning thirty, believing it was then or never, decided to have just one child. He concluded that his wife might well feel the same someday and prepared himself to face the question when and if it arose. Besides, he was curious to see what he'd want. His parents had had him—their only child—quite late. There was plenty of time.

Of one thing Jack and his wife were sure: not another abortion. She'd had it about a year after they married. Though quick and painless, apparently traumatic neither surgically nor psychologically, she was left feeling that she should have been more careful, that she'd forced herself into a set of choices she had no wish to make. Of course it was her body, she wasn't going to be a child-producing machine, she never really thought about not going through with it, but she was angry at herself for having created the beginning of a life only to terminate it. Bad business, she thought. Unnecessary.

Jack concurred in her decision to have the abortion, but without enthusiasm, though as they spoke of it the issue seemed ultimately practical. They didn't want a child just then, if at all; an abortion was merely minor surgery; the capacity to abort a fetus was, apparently, part of life. Still, Jack was unsettled. Of course, he told himself, there were peoples that practiced infanticide—had to, just to survive. And he'd seen too many unwanted children to believe that life was in and of itself sacred. Hell, the people at Zero Population Growth knew what they were talking about too. Even so, Jack was disturbed. Like his wife, he wished they'd been more careful. He made a kind of peace with himself when, leafing through a book on Indian myths, he read that once a given soul tries to enter this life, it perseveres until it succeeds.

Few people who knew Jack would have accused him of being sentimental about children, "dwarfs," as he often referred to them. If he saw no automatic virtue in parenting, so he reserved judgment on children, easily charmed by them but just as easily put off if they were spoiled or out of control. "Haywire," his mother had always said to describe him when he was confused or hysterical as an adolescent. He'd never liked the word, but could appreciate his mother's feeling now that he was an adult.

On the other hand, Jack was sometimes surprised. A couple he knew had a baby, and Jack predicted, correctly, that the husband would never change a diaper, never get up in the middle of the night if the baby cried. He could not have imagined, however, the child's beatific smiles of discovery and delight as she and her father pushed a beach ball back and forth. Nor did he foresee the compassion and vulnerability that emerged in his friend when the child became ill.

As he reached his mid-thirties, Jack's hungers for success were easing. He'd been making good money as a journalist for some time, had won several professional awards. His life was in order, he thought. Yet he found himself ever less interested in the flow of larger events. He'd interviewed too many politicians, been at the scene of too much mayhem, described too many wrongs. He was, finally, sick of the news. He began to spend more time at home, working in the garden, walking with his wife, building a toolshed, reading. These things were real, he thought. The rest was just a very intricate masquerade.

In this period Jack's father died. He'd had a long life, and a good one. Many people mourned his passing; for Jack the loss was assuaged by pride. As he measured the impact of his father's death, it registered on him that, neither of his parents having siblings, their bloodlines could end with him. He was too much a skeptic now to feel messianic about perpetuating himself through progeny, but he did feel that he'd just as soon not be the last of his particular kind.

Increasingly often, it seemed to him, the question of having children came up. A close friend had her second child twelve years after her first and, though cursing the endless diapers and sleepless nights, was clearly happy. A painter he knew married a woman with three children, worked hard to support his new family, gave up enormous amounts of the private time he'd for years so zealously protected. His life was richer now, he told Jack.

Another friend, a longtime bachelor, expressed the fear one

night that he'd pay for not having children, that he'd end up alone in some skid-row hotel. Was this, Jack wondered, an argument in favor of having children? To protect oneself emotionally, if not financially? He recalled that, fighting with his parents when he was thirteen, enraged, he'd asked why they'd had him. They were silent, Jack remembered, as if wondering themselves. Years had passed, but Jack still felt he was unwilling to risk a similar question from a child of his own. Or to have to respond that he'd just gone ahead and done it. What kind of answer would that be?

And then at a family reunion one of Jack's cousins asked him when he was going to have kids.

"Probably not for a while," Jack said, tossing off a quick answer to what seemed a perfunctory question.

"You're right," his cousin replied. "We had too many too fast. Never should have done it." Jack didn't know quite what to say. Finally, he asked his cousin why they did.

"Tell you the truth," his cousin said, "once we had the first, we figured why not the whole bunch."

"But why the first?"

"Well," his cousin answered, "I could tell you my wife wanted it, and she did. Then too, people expected us to have a family. That's the way it was. But even so, that doesn't explain what was going on. There was just some point when we decided to go ahead, both of us. A feeling, that's all. That's how it was."

For years Jack had worked hard to shape his life, to free himself of what might confine him. So many times, he thought, he could have been snared. What if he'd married his high-school sweetheart? And professionally Jack saw many of his colleagues just marking time, going through the motions, all he'd fought not to do. If he'd intuited early on that many things simply happen, nonetheless action, effort, making change had been his way. Yet now, gaining perspective on needs once so urgent, he began to feel that his younger self had been someone else entirely. Same name, same limbs and organs, but little more. Pulling out an old photograph of himself one night, he studied the twenty year old in the picture. Lean and hungry. Cocksure. His wife loved the picture, the black T-shirt, cigarette dangling from the lip, the James Dean/young Brando look, told Jack she wished she'd known him then. But for Jack the photograph was of someone else. He'd changed, had lost the illusion of having control of his life. And like his cousin, he thought, he was responding to feelings he could in no way justify. Not even to himself.

Feelings. Sifting through his life from time to time, Jack wondered if there was a thinness in the world he and his wife had built. He loved her more all the time, in part because he knew too well how easily things could be destroyed, in part in response to her deepening love for him. But was it not, he asked himself, affection that would have gone to their children? Did his wife not sense this? Was their home—so spare, so ordered—too immaculate? They had peace, but wasn't it in some way sterile? They ate no red meat, drank bottled water, took vitamins, got the best organic vegetables. Had they cared for themselves too well? So many questions; Jack was glad at least to be old enough not to expect immediate answers. If any. He'd just see what happened. What else was there? How could he have once believed he knew it all?

"I think I'm going to go ahead and apply to law school," his wife told him one morning at the breakfast table. She'd been thinking about it for nearly a year, tired of her part-time job as a commercial artist. She wanted power to influence things, she'd said several times, wanted to be able to affect the real world. Her ambition had more than once brought a wry smile to Jack's lips. Even as he felt that he'd just as soon never have to deal with that world again, his wife wanted to get further into it. The era of women, Jack thought, and he hoped they enjoyed their shot at opportunity and power. They couldn't do worse than men.

"Good," Jack said that morning. "Go ahead. I'll work for a few more years, expose some more bastards, and then I'll retire."

"To do what?" his wife responded, laughing. "You'll go crazy."

"No I won't," Jack said testily. "I'm changing. I'll find something. Maybe I'll just be a house-husband. Aren't they coming into vogue?"

"That won't be enough for you and you know it."

"It might, it might, particularly if we had kids."

"But we don't. Remember?"

"You're absolutely right," Jack said. "But anyway, you're going to law school."

"Wait a minute, not so fast. If you were going to be a house-husband, that might make things different. I wouldn't have to miss more than a semester to have a baby. It's not impossible."

"I'll keep that in mind," Jack replied, reaching over to kiss her. "Watch out."

The next morning he went to the public library. Looking under embryology in the card catalogue, he soon located a shelf of volumes dealing with conception, pregnancy, and birth. In one book, he saw incredible color photographs shot inside the womb, read that at eleven weeks the fetus "like an astronaut in his capsule . . . floats in its amniotic sac with the villi of the placenta around it like a radiant wreath." He was amazed to see the closed eyes of the fetus at five months, the "unearthly calm" of the face.

Picking up another book, he learned about the potential hazards of labor and about the trauma of birth—what the writers described as entry into the "kingdom of opposites." It was when Jack read that the child's first breath feels like fire, sears the lungs, that he decided he'd absorbed enough for one day.

In bed that night, his wife woke to find Jack sitting up against the headboard counting on his fingers.

"For the love of God," she said, "what are you doing?"

"Arithmetic. You made me lose count."

"Of what?"

"I'm trying to figure out what astrological sign a child conceived now would have."

"Well?"

"Wait a second. Okay. Scorpio."

"No thanks," his wife said. "No thanks."

"Why?"

"I don't know any Scorpios I like, that's all."

"Fair enough. How about Sagittarians?"

"Much better."

"Careful. I'll remember that in a few weeks."

"You be careful," she said, kissing him. "You're the one who'll end up changing diapers. Ca-ca."

"Ca-ca?"

"Absolutely right. Think it over, house-husband-to-be."

"I can't be scared," Jack said, grinning. "I'm a hard-bitten journalist. I've seen it all. A little crap isn't going to intimidate me."

"Whatever you say," his wife replied. "Now, if you don't mind I'm going back to sleep."

As Jack finally dozed off, right palm on his wife's belly, he was smiling. Not at the prospect of dirty diapers, it should be said. No, future coming into focus, he could just make out a recently conceived Sagittarian. One-fifth of an inch long. Sex not yet apparent. Vestigial gills. A tail. No more than a newt—and his, by God!—but taking shape, recapitulating the evolution of the phylum. Gaining strength. Preparing to be born.

Passion's Duration

You should have seen them when they first met. God, they couldn't get enough of each other, making love until all hours of the night, on the phone if separated for even several hours, thinking of each other whenever they passed beyond the reach of still another sweet embrace. This was, truly, the passion of which the poets sing.

Skeptics, rest easy; romantics, stand and be counted! Ponder this: sustained passion is similar to perpetual motion, a perfection inexorably denied by some almost negligible friction. Why talk of blame, character, choice? There are laws. We can even attempt the thermodynamic, something like, "Passion is inversely proportional to familiarity." (After an initial period of grace, of course.) Think of it. Perhaps passion, like other forms of energy, can be neither created nor destroyed. Merely found, and lost. Perhaps also this constant amount of passion in the atmosphere is not quite enough to go around, must therefore be kept moving for the benefit of the species as a whole. How else would people ever get together?

If such speculation seems too mechanistic, let us examine the facts. To begin with, our lovers so exhausted themselves in bed that one evening she suggested they sleep apart a night, just to get some rest. She put down several cushions on the living room floor, brought out another set of sheets, and was dreaming—of him—by the time her head hit the pillow she'd taken from the double bed. He, too, quickly fell asleep. But, waking several hours later, cold north wind shaking the windowpanes, he got up, shivering, and came into the living room. He told himself it was wrong to disturb her, yet, grinning to imagine himself Prince to her Sleeping Beauty, brushed her lips with his until she reached out for him. They woke, very late for work, utterly exhausted.

The next night they tried it again, but this time he promised to let her sleep. In the morning both felt better and made love with renewed vigor. Several days later, sensibly enough, they purchased a second mattress and springs. If they spent nights in the same bed, both agreed, their passion would utterly consume them.

How to calibrate change? This nocturnal separation was merely an attempt to be reasonable, an acknowledgment that there could be too much of a good thing. Led to nothing more serious than arguments about who would come to whose room to make love; who, passion spent, would have to traverse the ice-cold floor back to an unwarmed bed. No, though a bit odd, this arrangement was hardly remarkable, nothing to misconstrue. On the other hand, after they'd been together nearly a month he developed an allergic reaction to the hair of her blue-eyed Samoyed. His own eyes began to water if she embraced him without washing her hands after petting the dog. Sometimes, approaching him for a kiss, she'd realize that her hands weren't clean and would have to control her impulse. And, not surprisingly, sometimes she just didn't feel like washing her hands yet another time. He went to the doctor for shots, never blamed her or the dog, but there it was, a small impediment to the direct flow of feeling. A little something between them.

Though their passion continued unabated, a constant miracle they created together, there were several other minor problems. She complained that he failed to clean the dishes carefully when he washed them. After starting to protest once that no one else had ever mentioned it, he caught himself, smiled, and promised to be more thorough. Meanwhile, he found that he didn't much care for her closest friend, who seemed to him to be displeased that they were living together. He even got into the habit of going out "on errands" when the friend came by. Though he never mentioned it, he was irritated by feeling compelled to leave his own house. But, of course, he'd been the one who'd insisted that she give up her apartment.

None of these problems, really, affected the great desire they had for each other. In this period, however, having experienced a series of debilitating stomach ailments (which, she noted, began right after she moved in with him), she decided to go on a strict organic and meatless diet. For nearly a week he shared her new regimen, eating large salads, much fruit, tofu, and various kinds of nuts, but then announced one evening that he'd bought a steak. Sitting alone at the dining room table after he'd broiled it, he ate with pleasure and noisily drank the juice from his plate.

That night he also told her that organic produce was just too expensive. Soon, accordingly, they purchased their food at different stores to prepare separate dinners. Initially, one cooked and then waited for the other to do the same so that they could dine together. But sometimes one of them had an appointment or a class in the evening, and, kitchen so small, the process of making two dinners took time. Before long they often ate separately. Further, she'd found that the sight of raw meat now made her nauseous, that even the smell was more than she could bear. Trying to be considerate, she said nothing, but of course he noticed that she'd come into the kitchen when he was cooking to throw the windows wide open.

In the ensuing weeks she purchased a number of books on organic diets and pored over them, occasionally explaining to him, for instance, the mucus-inducing potential of the foods he consumed. He was more sarcastic than he intended one night when he told her that even if organic food was becoming her metaphysic, he preferred to be an agnostic, if need be even to have his soul end up in some char-broiled hell. Sensing immediately that he'd gone too far, he tried to retreat to the solid terrain of fact, and pointed out that she still drank countless cups of coffee each day and smoked cigarettes. If he thought that demonstrating an anomaly would stave off her anger, however, he was sadly mistaken.

Her smoking was in fact a real problem for them. He'd stopped five years before, after a tremendous ordeal of depression and what he remembered as near insanity. He'd actually told himself before meeting her that he'd never live with a woman who smoked. The sad truth being that he still yearned for a cigarette and didn't need the stress of constant temptation. He finally asked her not to smoke in the house but relented when the winter rains came. Instead, he posted a no-smoking sign on his bedroom door and kept it closed all day.

She told him she understood, even tried to cut down on her smoking, but something about the closed door exasperated her. Often he'd return from work and, an avid reader, would stay in his room with a book for hours, keeping out of the living room both because she smoked there and because her Samoyed liked to curl up on the sofa. Sometimes, looking down the hall toward his bedroom door, she couldn't help feeling that he was closing her out.

The problem of her cigarettes was finally solved, after a fashion, when he began to smoke again. Soon he was up to more than two packs a day, while she found that her own consumption quickly doubled. Feeling pains in his legs and chest, he couldn't stop himself from blaming her; while she, now suffering from a hacking cough, insisted that until he began again she'd always smoked in moderation. Every few days he'd try to quit, growing more irritable as the hours without a cigarette passed, until, seeing her light up, he'd grab the pack, glaring at her.

Could anything else, one wonders, come between them? Well, yes. She frequently suffered from insomnia, while he had an obsession about burglars. Often her restless pacing in the middle of the night would snap him out of a deep sleep, his hand groping in the dark for the can of Mace he kept by his bed. Worse, perhaps, he played the flute. Badly. An accomplished pianist, she not only quickly abandoned the idea of accompanying him, but grew to dread his practicing, the same mistakes repeated over and over again. Finally, her checks often bounced. If she thought nothing of it, he, coming from a poor family, had grown up forever in shame about the dunning of creditors. He knew it was none of his business, but just to see her leafing absentmindedly through a stack of unpaid bills set his teeth on edge.

What, then, of their passion? Strange as it may seem, even after bitter argument they could sometimes work their way back to each other by making love. By this time, of course, it was quite different than when they met. So much to ignore; so much to forget; such deep breaths to take simply to exhale the rage. Just to decide who would come to whose room required careful negotiation and diplomacy: someone had to concede. And even then her hands had to be washed clean of the Samoyed, he had to brush his teeth to eliminate the smell of cooked flesh. Nonetheless, on rare occasions, so much dangerous terrain finally spanned, their loving would be almost sweeter than before. Tinged, now, with the fear of loss; with self-reproach; and, in the small hours of the night, once in a very great while, with a piquant sadness for all that had come between them.

Mad Dog, One More Time

No, these were hardly high times. Chain letters and pyramid schemes proliferated; money, various entrepreneurs said, was love. The bodies of Reverend Jones and his followers were finally tallied and shipped home from Guyana. Coca-Cola established an exclusive contract with China, and Chinese technocrats arrived in the United States to see what we had to sell. A new market, almost a billion potential consumers: new hope for our way of life. Weapons for oil; straight business. So much for Mao.

Late one autumn afternoon, nearly a year after he'd piped the pimp and left for Reno and points east, Mad Dog wheeled his battered VW bug up my driveway. It turned out that he and his "wife"—though he frequently used the word, I gathered that no clerk or cleric had tampered with their vows—were already settled in town. She'd found work in a fabric store, while he'd come up with a job in an auto repair shop. He was learning a lot, he told me, and had even arranged to be paid under the table. No withholding, no retirement, and, declaring no income, he could still draw his monthly check from the state for being a basket case. What with his medical benefits and food stamps, they were already setting money aside to buy land up north.

Scams notwithstanding, Mad Dog was genuinely pleased to be working again, had cut down to six beers a day, and looked fine.

A sergeant perennially searching for the right army, Mad Dog respected his new boss and was determined to do a better job than anyone could have asked. This was quintessential Mad Dog, playing a strong supporting role in some World War II movie that never stopped running in his mind's eye. Given half a chance, he'd be the tough bastard who always chewed everyone out but who then used his body to smother the live grenade, saving his buddies by sacrificing himself.

If I was pleased to find Mad Dog looking good, I was particularly glad to see him because I'd been playing a lot of basketball. When we reached the court that afternoon, he was duly impressed with how much I'd improved, and I felt that my labors in life had not been entirely without reward.

During the past year I'd not only learned more about basketball but had come to know the regulars on the court, though it had taken me several months to get used to spotting them around town in street clothes, to believe that they actually had lives outside the game. They'd stare at me, too, as if, not wearing my shorts and high-top sneakers, I was in costume. If I saw them when I was with my wife, I'd notice them appraising her, perhaps wondering how a 25 percent outside shooter could score so well in the game of love.

Spending so much time playing basketball, I found that having to wait for another turn when my team lost became less onerous. The men in line to play would sit on the side of the court against the wall, catching the weak warmth of the setting sun. Resting, loosening up, maybe taking hits off a joint, they'd hoot when someone on the court was beaten badly, laugh when a prayer shot dropped in, applaud a fine move, jeer when a player they disliked was shooting well. What a different sport it was from the sideline! How obvious the mistakes, how manifest the hungers. A man would make an incredible shot, one the gods might never grant him again, and show no expression, as if nothing could be more normal, more true to his capacities. Players on the sideline would cackle.

Always there was talk, this other level of the game. If you played well you wanted to savor the moment, to get others to relive it with you before, so ephemeral, it was gone forever. If you looked bad, you wanted to be sure to let everyone know that you were just coming off the flu, that you hadn't played for three weeks, that your bad heel was acting up. And, finally, since everyone on the court periodically lost his temper, argued maniacally over nothing, played the prima donna, just plain blew it, talking it over was not only a search for concurrence but a form of apology. No one was ever right enough to stay silent for long.

The talk: stories, character analysis, apologias. Subjects of interest included why Big D always called out the score incorrectly (and in his favor); why Danny shot so much even when he was missing; how Lonnie managed to keep the game so free of argument when he played. Nor were matters beyond the court off limits. Why did Rick Barry pout? Was *Invasion of the Body Snatchers* as good as *Carrie?* Would the Warriors get Bill Walton? Couldn't the deaths in Guyana have been averted if Reverend Jones had been into basketball? The sideline consensus on this point was that the game would have turned Jones's paranoia to nothing worse than what we all experienced: occasional rage and an endless desire to run it again. If power was what Jones had wanted, after all, nothing could compare to looking good at pickup ball. And as for killing himself, well, it was widely understood that no one had ever willingly stopped playing the game.

There was the story, often recalled, of the player who sold forged football tickets to all the regulars, and no doubt made a nice piece of change at his hustle. But he then had to stay away from the court. What a price he paid.

As it turns out, Mad Dog became one of the sideline regulars' great topics of discussion. This is how it happened. He'd been working long hours, but generally managed to get up to the game just before nightfall, usually polishing off a beer as he arrived, often exhausted, sometimes drunk. More than once, when he seemed to forget to play defense, his teammates would get on him, but Mad Dog would just laugh or, smiling, tell them to fuck themselves. He was feeling good, working; the game just wasn't going to get to him, even if he messed it up for others.

Going to work one morning, he showed up at seven as usual to open the shop. He liked being there alone for a while each day, was flattered that his boss trusted him with the keys. When the parts man arrived on time at seven-thirty, Mad Dog took his normal break for his first cup of coffee. A few minutes later, as always, he realized that he'd better get to a toilet quick. That's just the way his system worked.

When Mad Dog asked for the key to the bathroom, the parts man started to pass it to him but then dangled it just beyond reach. Mad Dog didn't much like the game, feeling as though his sphincter would give way at any moment, so he told the parts man to stop fucking around. When Mad Dog reached for the key again, the parts man slapped his hand away. A big man, he'd been on Mad Dog's nerves for some time, always giving him a hard tap on the shoulder when he passed, just playing, of course, but treating Mad Dog as if it were clear that he could push him around.

"Look, asshole," Mad Dog finally said. "If you don't give me the key I'm going to split your fuckin' head open."

"Try it, sucker," the parts man responded.

Mad Dog didn't want to blow his job, but he had to have the key. What was he going to do, shit in his pants? He gave it one more try, hoping to shine the parts man on. "C'mon," he said, "enough's enough. Give me a break. I gotta go real bad."

"Tough titty," the parts man said, and laughed. He was still laughing as Mad Dog gave him a kick that shattered his kneecap. Then Mad Dog hauled him to his feet, broke his nose with a judo chop, dropped him, and picked up the key. Mad Dog was crying: he knew his boss would be upset by the violence, would see no percentage in keeping him around.

Mad Dog was half drunk when he showed up at the court that afternoon, and really hurting, feeling that he'd betrayed his boss, mourning the respect and affection that he'd lost. It was a strange day even before he arrived: too many men waiting for their turn, tempers flaring on the court, the action rough and sloppy. When Mad Dog finally got his game there were repeated arguments, but he just waited each one out, saying nothing. He played listlessly, without heart.

Over on the sideline we were talking, as usual, when the fight began. Big D threw a punch at Mad Dog and drew first blood. Apparently they'd collided with each other, hard. Already enraged by the arguments, and having missed all his shots, Big D decided to take it out on someone. He and Mad Dog had exchanged words before.

Giving away eight inches and fifty pounds, too drunk for strategy, Mad Dog stood toe to toe with Big D. They traded punches fast and furious, but Mad Dog couldn't get anything past Big D's long arms, and kept taking shots to the head and chest.

Both because most of the payers had no use for either man, and because all the evil of the day seemed to be working itself out in their combat, no one made a move to break it up, no one said a word.

Finally Mad Dog stepped back, shook his head a few times as though stopping himself from saying something, and then walked off the court toward his car. Catching up with him, I checked his cuts, but, blood aside, he was okay. I was more concerned with keeping him from getting a pipe or some Mace and coming back to settle with Big D. "Don't sweat it," Mad Dog said. "I'm not going to do a fuckin' thing. If I get him now they'll be twenty witnesses to assault with a deadly weapon. I'd get sent away forever. I had my shot at him but was too loaded to bring him down. You lose a fight every once in a while. That's just the way it is."

The game resumed that day, everyone quiet, chastened by the fight, seeing in it the worst of what they themselves so often expressed on the court. Big D showed up again the next afternoon, apparently without understanding that his life had been spared through no fault of his own, but Mad Dog stayed away. Job gone, game gone, he drank himself silly the next few weeks. Then one day I got a call from his wife. Mad Dog was in jail, arrested for shoplifting a pair of pants at a suburban shopping mall; the bail was five hundred dollars. Weeping at the appropriate moments, his wife conned a bondsman into putting up the money, though she must have known that Mad Dog had no intention of ever showing up in court. A convicted felon, he'd face a "petty with a prior," would stand to do real time even for a fourteen-dollar pair of pants.

Mad Dog knew it was time to go. This would be the fourth state he was wanted in, but, he laughed, there were plenty still to go. Warning him not to run through them too fast, I watched his VW bug pull off into the night. I haven't heard from him since.

The day after Christmas that year I shot better than 80 percent for five straight games. The next afternoon, sad to say, I was back to normal. Players who had seen my moment soon forgot it, and I had no proof for those who hadn't been there. What could I do but keep playing? Winter continued, but even on the cold gray days, whenever it didn't rain, I changed into my basketball gear, pulled on two pairs of sweat socks, laced up my high tops, and headed for the court. Of course the game went on.